IN PURSUIT OF PARENTHOOD

IN PURSUIT OF PARENTHOOD

Experiences of IVF

Kate Brian

Medical adviser: Richard J S Howell, BSC FRCOG
Consultant Obstetrician and Gynaecologist,
Homerton Hospital

BLOOMSBURY

To Max and Alfred

First published in Great Britain 1998
Bloomsbury Publishing Plc, 38 Soho Square, London W1V 5DF

Copyright © 1998 by Kate Brian

The moral right of the author has been asserted

A CIP catalogue record for this book
is available from the British Library

ISBN 0 7475 3747 X

10 9 8 7 6 5 4 3 2 1

Typeset by Hewer Text Ltd, Edinburgh
Printed in Great Britain by Clays Limited, St Ives plc

Contents

Acknowledgements

This book could not have been written without Sarah and Paul, Debbie and Tom, Katie and Michael, Tony and Claire, Jane and Mark, Polly and Marcus, Helen and Darryl, Hayley and Claude and Jackie and Nicky. It is as much their book as mine, and I cannot thank them enough.

I'm grateful to all the others who gave their time to talk to me at length about their experiences of IVF. Although their stories may not appear in the book, they were a source of inspiration and ideas.

I'd like to thank Richard Howell for his invaluable advice and suggestions, and Professor Peter Braude, Tim Hedgely of ISSUE and Barney Wyld at the HFEA for their help. I'm indebted to Jane McNeil for believing I could do this, and to Gil McNeil for her enthusiasm. I'd also like to thank Diana Tyler, Kate Bouverie, Kate Morris, Esther Jagger, Rosemary Davidson and everyone at Bloomsbury.

I am also grateful to all my family, friends and colleagues for their support not only during the writing of this book, but more importantly during the IVF itself. Special thanks to Anna McCord, Christine Oldfield, Tanya Sillem, Lucia Tambini and Jessica Rowan. My mother, Daphne McCord, helped more than she could possibly imagine.

Most of all my thanks and love to Max, and to Alfred who has made the world a much nicer place.

Foreword

Childlessness is only really appreciated by those who experience it. Couples who have difficulty in conceiving often feel lonely, shunned and isolated, too frightened or embarrassed to disclose, let alone to discuss the pain that they feel. They are often unsure how to go about getting more information about their disorder and what its treatment may entail. Gathering reliable information can be difficult and fact has to be sifted from salesmanship since the lack of funding for IVF or in vitro fertilisation within the National Health Service in this country has forced it predominantly into the private sector. As the subject of one of the case histories in this book says, 'Infertility is an industry . . . founded on hope . . . you are sold this fantasy that you're going to do it and it's going to work.'

Kate Brian uses her own story to lay out clearly and sympathetically each step of the investigative and treatment procedures, in a way that only someone who has experienced at first hand the frustrations and rigours required of a couple going through IVF can do. Each of the stories that she has gathered poignantly and pertinently gives clear insight into the pain and feelings of hopelessness that all too often go hand in hand with having to resort to IVF in the hope of having that desperately wanted child. Their revelations, their disappointments, and their joy when fortunate, make compelling reading. Here at last is a book by those who know what it is really like, written for couples who wish and need to understand.

However, it is more than just that – it is also a sad indictment of the way that some coupless are so insensitively handled by my own profession. Thus not only is this book a must for those seeking information about IVF; it is a must for every professional involved in the practice of IVF, a learning exercise that couldn't be more competently or clearly delivered.

Peter Braude MA PhD FRCOG
Professor and Chairman of the Division of Women and Children's Health, Guy's, King's and St Thomas's Medical Schools, and Director of Fertility Services, Guy's and St Thomas's Hospital Trust

Introduction

When I was first told I might have to consider IVF in order to have the baby I'd been longing for, I was terrified and wanted to know as much as I could about what would be involved. I read every book I could find on the subject and became extremely well versed in the mechanics of the process, but I still felt I didn't have any idea what IVF would be like for me as a patient. Even the books about infertility which had been written by people who had experienced treatment seemed to concentrate on explaining the medical procedures, and these had already been adequately explained by the staff at the clinic where I was being treated.

What I desperately wanted to know was how I would feel. Would I be able to go to work while I was having IVF? Was it best to tell your friends or to keep it a secret? Was it really possible to do the injections yourself? Would the drugs make me feel dreadful? Would it hurt when they took the eggs out? Later, once I started the treatment cycle I was longing to know how other people dealt with it. Was it normal to feel this way? Did everyone find it so lonely? Was I taking it all too seriously or did other women get elated or depressed at every scan? The stress and anxiety of waiting to find out whether it had worked, the devastating effect of an unsuccessful treatment cycle and the elation of success after so many years of disappointment are all part of an overwhelming experience which nothing has prepared you for.

This book is an attempt to answer some of the questions I had, and is for anyone who is going through IVF or who thinks they may do so in the future. It is also for their friends and relatives, and anyone else who wants to understand what is involved for prospective parents in the making of a test-tube baby.

It doesn't go through the procedures of in vitro fertilisation in great medical detail. Instead it aims to give a basic guide to IVF, explaining the stages of treatment from the patient's point of view and discussing the emotions which may arise as the cycle progresses. I've used my experiences to illustrate this, and those of nine other couples who tell their own stories. In the course of writing the book I spoke to many more, and discussed with them all the things they wished someone had told them before they embarked on their first IVF cycles. I have endeavoured to make sure those gaps have been filled, and to give as wide a picture as possible of what IVF may be like.

Obviously, every treatment cycle is different and it would never be possible to cover every situation or outcome. There may still be a lot to be learnt from seeing how other people have dealt with their personal situations, and indeed just from knowing that you are not alone. The pain of not being able to have a child when you long for one is something no one can understand unless they have experienced it themselves. Those of us who have know exactly what it is like, and we hope our stories might make it hurt a little less for you.

1

The Route to IVF

The women of today's child-bearing generation are used to being in control of their own lives. We make our own decisions about what we want to do, and when we want to do it. We have grown up with readily available contraception which has allowed us to take charge of our fertility, leaving the decision about when or whether to have children entirely in our hands. It has sometimes seemed so straightforward to prevent ourselves conceiving that we have assumed it will be just as easy to allow ourselves to get pregnant. The realisation that it might not be possible to have a baby when we want to can come as a great shock.

The desire for a child is so fundamental and instinctive that we can't always explain our feelings of failure and loss when it remains unfulfilled. So much of our day-to-day living is interwoven with the expectation that once we find a partner and settle down we will reproduce and have a family. There are constant painful reminders of our failure, which is not easy for the happily fertile majority to comprehend. Infertility can be an isolating experience and everyday situations may become difficult to deal with. Innocent enquiries as to whether you have children, a friend telling you she is pregnant again, or a visit to see a newborn baby can leave you wretched, and hating yourself for feeling so bitter.

I was thirty when I started trying to conceive. I'd always known I'd like to have children one day, but it seemed important to have a career and sort out the rest of my life first. Finally my partner, Max, and I decided the time was right, so we threw away the contraceptives and hoped I'd be pregnant within a few months. I had sometimes thought how terrible it would be to discover you couldn't have children. Infertility had seemed a dark and frightening affliction, something people mentioned in hushed, embarrassed tones, and those who suffered it were rather tragic figures.

After some months of not getting pregnant, I met a woman who told me she was having problems conceiving a third child and was taking fertility drugs which were 'all but guaranteed' to get you pregnant. Soon afterwards I decided to see whether my GP could shed any light on my failure to conceive. I was hoping he would assure me there was nothing wrong, but I couldn't help thinking that it might be useful to get hold of some of this woman's wonderful fertility drugs and solve the problem immediately. In fact I never discovered what she was taking, but I did find out that there's absolutely nothing which can 'all but guarantee' to get you pregnant, and it didn't take me long to realise that there are no easy answers or quick solutions when it comes to fertility.

IVF, or in vitro fertilisation, is often heralded as the miraculous solution to all our fertility problems. Everyone seems to know someone who has had a test-tube baby, in the same way that everyone knows a couple who tried to have a baby for fifteen years and then conceived unexpectedly on the day they were accepted as parents by an adoption agency. The publicity and hype surrounding IVF can lead you to imagine that you should rush off to a clinic and demand it the moment you suspect you have a problem, but it is likely to be some time before you reach the point where doctors decide it may be the best way forward for you. Most couples who have IVF will have spent years going through tests and other treatments first. Once IVF has been suggested there is often more time spent on a waiting list before the treatment can start.

The route to IVF can be long, difficult and lonely, but it is a well-trodden path. There has been a steady rise in the number of couples opting for treatment, with around thirty thousand treatment cycles carried out each year in the United Kingdom alone. The success rates, sometimes called the 'take home baby' rates, have also been rising to reflect advances in techniques, and currently stand at about 15 per cent per treatment cycle started.

Many people are surprised to discover that a treatment which is so much discussed offers such a low chance of success, and the reality is that the vast majority of couples will not find an instant answer to their fertility problems with their first attempt at IVF. Cumulative success rates are slightly more cheering, suggesting that up to 70 per cent of couples will succeed over four or more treatment cycles. The one question everyone considering IVF wants answered is whether the treatment will work for them eventually, but that's something no one can answer with any certainty. The prognosis is better for women under forty and for couples where the man has a normal sperm count, but despite all the medical advances in assisted conception doctors still can't always explain why some treatment cycles work and others don't.

Society's attitudes to infertility can seem harsh and uncaring, with little in the way of help and support for those who aren't finding it easy to have a child of their own. People who have had children without any problems may talk glibly about infertility as nature's way of preventing overpopulation; they tell you they don't 'agree' with IVF, which they may see as an unnatural meddling with nature. Infertile couples, and women in particular, are often portrayed as desperate, slightly unhinged people who will stop at nothing to get the child they long for. There is much debate about the current climate, in which most people pay for their treatment; some critics of the system feel that infertile couples are viewing babies as part of a lifestyle package they can purchase in the same way that they might buy a house or a new car. Many a fertile commentator is happy to hold forth on the moral wrongs of the concept of the 'right to a baby', which they seem to believe is the way those of us who can't get pregnant without help think about it. In fact, all that most couples dare to hope is that their treatment might give them the opportunity to have a child. The idea of the 'right to a baby' is firmly rooted only in the minds of the fertile.

Infertility is often misunderstood, partly because many people who have had to endure it find it too painful to talk about. Sharing the experiences of others, and knowing that you are not the only ones to live through what can sometimes seem like a ghastly nightmare, is one way of making it hurt a little less.

SEEING YOUR DOCTOR

There are no hard and fast rules about how long you should try to get pregnant before you see a doctor. On average a fertile couple will take at least three or four months to conceive, but it is perfectly normal for it to take much longer and most doctors advise waiting a year or more before you seek medical help. However, a lot depends on your individual situation and your age.

Women become less fertile as they get older and, whilst an older woman may take longer to conceive, she is likely to be more aware of her biological clock ticking away. If you are over thirty-five it is worth seeing a doctor sooner rather than later. The same applies for a woman who has had any previous pelvic infections or cervical problems, or has problems with her periods. For men, problems with the testicles or previous sexual infections can be relevant. The best way to decide when to seek medical help with conception is to follow your own feelings. You will know when you are ready to talk to a doctor.

ASSESSING YOUR SITUATION

The first thing the doctor will need to know is how long you have been trying to conceive. It is not uncommon for people to be tempted to lie about this, feeling that they won't be taken seriously unless they have been trying for, say, two years; but it isn't a good idea, as it means your doctor won't have a true picture of your situation. Most will accept that something which has become a problem for you deserves to be taken seriously.

I felt very anxious when I first went to my GP, as I quite expected him to be unsympathetic and to tell me to go away and come back when we'd been trying for a few years. In fact he was immediately very reassuring and explained how common the problem is. One in six couples have difficulty conceiving, but we are often not aware of those around us who are in the same situation because it is something we tend to keep to ourselves. You should remember that you are most unlikely to be the first person your GP has seen who has concerns about not being able to conceive.

The doctor will want to see both partners and to check your medical history for anything which could be an obvious cause of the problem. A basic physical examination may also be helpful at this stage. The GP may carry out some tests straightaway, or may refer you to a specialist.

WHAT COULD BE WRONG

The first thing any tests will try to establish is the reason for the problem. There is no single cause of infertility, and getting through all the tests can be a lengthy process, as there are a number of possibilities which need to be eliminated.

When the reproductive process is working well, every month a woman's ovaries produce an egg which will travel down her fallopian tubes towards the uterus. Sperm produced by the man during intercourse meets the egg in the tubes and fertilises it. The fertilised egg will grow into an embryo, and implant in the womb. A problem at any stage in the procedure in either partner can prevent conception from taking place.

For the man, the problem most often lies with the sperm and may be attributed to physical or hormonal complications. Environmental factors may also play a role, as smoking and alcohol can both affect sperm. The sperm count may be low, which means there are less sperm than usual found in the semen, and there may be problems with the sperm quality. For instance, the sperm may not be moving about very well or they might have some kind of abnormality. Sometimes there are no sperm present in the semen at all.

There are more potential problem areas for a woman, which means she will usually end up having more tests than her male partner. One of the first things to check is whether she is producing eggs, or ovulating. Hormonal problems can be the cause when a woman isn't ovulating, and may be helped by drugs to stimulate the ovaries. In some cases the failure to ovulate may be due to a premature menopause which has caused egg production to stop, and in such situations it would be necessary to consider using eggs from a donor.

Endometriosis, a common condition where the cells which normally line the womb are found growing elsewhere in the body, can also affect fertility as it may damage the fallopian tubes or ovaries and can cause adhesions. Any kind of damage to the ovaries, tubes, womb or cervix may contribute to a fertility problem, whether the damage is congenital or caused by a previous illness or infection.

Polycystic ovary syndrome is another possible problem for women. As many as one in five women have small cysts on their ovaries which can be detected by ultrasound scan. For the majority they don't cause any problems. However, in some cases they can affect hormone production, and ovulation may become irregular or stop altogether. This is known as polycystic ovary syndrome. Fertility drugs to induce ovulation may be prescribed for a woman with polycystic ovary syndrome who is trying to get pregnant.

In a surprisingly high number of patients who seek help and undergo tests, no reason will be found for their failure to conceive. Up to a quarter of patients will be told that their infertility is unexplained, although this will probably be reduced to about 15 per cent once exhaustive tests have been carried out. If no cause can be found doctors may suggest that you wait a while before undergoing any kind of treatment, particularly if you are still reasonably young and have not been trying to conceive for too long. Some couples may welcome this as an opportunity to have a break and forget about medical investigations and intervention for a while, but for others it can be hard to accept once they have started to try to find a solution to their problem.

My partner and I found it quite frustrating not to know why we couldn't have a child. Max was convinced I would get pregnant eventually if we left it to nature, but I was much less optimistic and was certain there must be a cause which the doctors hadn't been able to discover. The most difficult thing about unexplained infertility is that well-meaning friends are always eager to assure you that you could probably get pregnant if you were relaxed enough, went on holiday, gave up trying and so on.

TEMPERATURE CHARTS

My doctor's first suggestion was that I should try keeping a temperature chart for a few months, which is meant to help a woman check that she is producing eggs. The temperature should rise slightly after ovulation, when the egg leaves the ovary, and by plotting your temperature on a chart every day you should start to see when this happens. A temperature chart can also help you to become familiar with your individual cycle, and to make sure you know when you are most likely to become pregnant, which is around the time of ovulation. In a regular 28-day cycle, ovulation normally occurs around day 14.

Some women find temperature charts very helpful, but I was firmly in the group of those who don't. Having gone out and bought a thermometer specially for the purpose and dutifully taken my temperature every morning for a couple of months, I was most distressed to find it remaining at exactly the same level throughout. I decided there must be something wrong with the thermometer, so I went and bought a more expensive model and started marking the daily reading on a chart. Although there was an occasional rise or fall, it bore no resemblance to the neat peaks I'd seen in the sample fertility charts in books where you could identify precisely when ovulation was occurring. It was only after I'd convinced myself that I didn't have any eggs at all that I discovered it is possible to be ovulating normally and not notice any rise in temperature.

It is worth trying to keep a temperature chart if your GP suggests it, but it is certainly not worth worrying if it proves a fruitless exercise. Although a chart may help you establish the pattern of your menstrual cycle, you can do this much more easily by keeping a simple record of menstruation over a few months. All you have to do is record the number of days in each cycle, counting from the first day of one period to the first day of the next. By monitoring this over a few months you will quickly get an idea of your individual cycle.

Even if your temperature chart does seem to be showing that you are ovulating, it may not help pinpoint your optimum chance of getting pregnant, as the most fertile time is just before and during ovulation, and therefore just before the change in temperature, although it is of course possible to get pregnant by having intercourse soon after ovulation.

OVULATION PREDICTION KITS

These kits are a rather more sophisticated way of plotting your cycle. They are widely available at chemists and can even be found on some supermarket shelves. Using a urine dipstick, you can monitor your hormone levels and find out when you are about to ovulate. They may be helpful but can give misleading readings, and as they are expensive you may not want to use them for months on end to try to ensure you are having intercourse at the optimum time.

REFERRAL TO A SPECIALIST

It is probably advantageous to be referred to a specialist fertility unit for tests early in the investigation period. Initially I was referred to the gynaecology department at my local hospital, as the waiting time for an appointment there was considerably less than the six months to see a consultant at the nearest fertility clinic. We thought we could find the cause of the problem more quickly by going to the local hospital, but in retrospect this was a mistake. After more than a year of inconclusive tests and unsuccessful treatment at the local hospital I was referred to the fertility unit, and then had to wait six months for an appointment at a time when I was much more desperate and upset.

Treatment at a specialist unit will not only be more expert and thorough, it is usually more sympathetic. At a local hospital's gynaecology department, on the other hand, you will often be seen in a general clinic session and not with others who are experiencing fertility problems. Tests may need to be repeated later if you end up going to a specialist unit, as many specialists prefer to work from their own more detailed assessments. The emphasis will be on the female partner, and men may feel uncomfortable in an atmosphere where the priority is 'women's problems'. None of the doctors I saw at the local hospital ever expressed any interest in seeing or talking to Max. When he came with me to appointments he was left sitting outside in the waiting room while I saw the doctor. When we did insist that we both went in to see the doctor he was often completely ignored and felt very left out. Our failure to conceive was always discussed as my problem, although no cause had been found. In fact it was only after we had been trying to have a child for more than two years that anyone bothered to give Max a physical examination.

At the local hospital I saw a succession of junior doctors who invariably spent most of the appointment time trying to find things in my notes, and sometimes seemed to know very little about fertility. The most peculiar appointment was with a young female doctor who was clearly confused by the fact that no one had found a reason for our failure to conceive. 'Did you know,' she said, leaning across her desk conspiratorially, 'that you are more likely to get pregnant at certain times in your monthly cycle than at others?' When I said I did know this, she looked rather disappointed and flicked her way through my notes again before coming up with another suggestion. 'Are you sure you aren't using contraceptives?' she asked with a slightly desperate air. This after a year and a half of failing to conceive! When I said I was quite certain she decided she would have to ask the consultant what to do next, and disappeared for the rest of my appointment time. She returned briefly to say I should come back in a few weeks for some more tests.

THE SPERM TEST

One of the first tests to be carried out is a sperm test. The man has to give a semen sample which is analysed in a laboratory to check the volume, the number of sperm present and their quality. The clinic may ask you to abstain from intercourse for two or three days before the sample is produced. Some men find the whole idea rather threatening at first, and it is particularly daunting if the sample has to be produced at the clinic or hospital. Some clinics have special rooms for the purpose and provide magazines or even videos for the occasion, but at a surprising number men are expected to make do in the toilets.

If you live relatively close to the clinic it should be possible to produce a sample at home and take it there immediately. You should be given instructions and a little pot to contain the sample, which will be marked with your name and the date and time at which it was produced. You will need to get it back within a set time, usually a maximum of a couple of hours. It is important that the sample is fresh as the motility, or movement, of the sperm will decrease with time. A fresh sample is needed to give an accurate reading of the number of sperm and their quality.

The sperm test should be repeated, because the results can be misleading and may change from day to day. A man who is perfectly fertile may, for instance, produce a sample with a low count from time to time. Ideally there should be two tests which are carried out at least a month apart. The analysis at a specialist fertility clinic tends to be more detailed than that at a general hospital. Even when no male problem is found, the male partner will rapidly lose any qualms about the sperm test as it becomes a routine part of fertility treatment.

BLOOD TESTS

For the woman, the first tests will usually be blood tests to check that her hormone levels are normal. The level of the hormone progesterone increases after an egg has been released, and by checking the amount in the blood doctors can get an indication of whether she is ovulating. Progesterone levels peak about seven days after ovulation, which in a regular (twenty-eight-day) cycle will tend to be twenty-one days after the start of a period. However, the results can be misleading if your cycle is irregular, longer or shorter. The blood tests may have to be repeated to fit your individual pattern.

If a woman has irregular periods, a full hormonal evaluation will be done and blood tests will be used to assess the levels of pituitary and thyroid hormones. Blood tests may also be used to check prolactin levels. Prolactin is a hormone which is produced when breastfeeding, and it can prevent you from ovulating if the levels are high.

When they do the blood tests clinics usually take the opportunity to check for rubella immunity, as rubella can be dangerous in pregnancy. If you don't have rubella immunity you would be advised to have a vaccination before starting treatment. (This would usually be done by a GP.)

ULTRASOUND SCAN

Clinics use ultrasound to check that the ovaries look normal and to give an indication of whether ovulation is taking place, as it should be possible to see on the scan the follicles in which eggs are produced. Scans may be carried out by placing the scanner on the abdomen, or by using a vaginal probe. It is a completely painless procedure whichever way it is done; however, with the abdominal scan you may have to drink several pints of water beforehand, as the soundwaves used travel best through fluid and produce a clearer picture if the bladder is full. It can be incredibly uncomfortable to have to sit in a hospital waiting room feeling as if you are about to burst, and it always seems to happen on the day when the clinic is running very late and you have to wait way past your appointment time.

THE POST-COITAL TEST

The post-coital test is one of the most unromantic procedures carried out in fertility investigations. It is used to make sure that the sperm are surviving in the cervical mucus. You are told to have intercourse at a certain time of day before going to the hospital. A sample of mucus is taken from the cervix during an internal examination and examined under a microscope to make sure the sperm are alive and swimming about.

If the test is negative and the sperm are dead it doesn't necessarily mean that your cervical mucus is killing your part-ner's sperm. It may be that the investigation has been done at the wrong time of the month, or that there is a problem with the sperm on that particular day. The test may be repeated if the results are negative or inconclusive.

The actual procedure is very much like a smear test and is completely painless, but I felt there was something demoralising and very intrusive about it. It's one thing to have to have intercourse on a particular day to try to conceive, but to have to have sex at a particular time on a particular day and then go dashing off to the hospital is a depressing corroboration of your failure to conceive. Fortunately, many clinics are now question-ing the value of the post-coital test.

LAPAROSCOPY

The most invasive female test is laparoscopy, which is used to examine the fallopian tubes and ovaries. It will show up any abnormalities or adhesions, and will also reveal any endometriosis. It is a fairly straightforward operation, done under general anaesthetic. A small incision is made in the navel and the stomach is inflated with carbon dioxide to allow a good view of the pelvic organs. Then a tiny telescope is inserted to let the medical team see what is happening inside. Dye is passed through the fallopian tubes to make sure they are clear, or patent. Most clinics now do laparoscopy on a day-care basis, which means you can go home a few hours after the operation, but others require an overnight stay in hospital.

I had never had any kind of operation before, and was quite scared by the prospect of a laparoscopy. Cutting me open seemed a rather extreme way of checking whether there was a problem, and I questioned whether it was necessary. In fact laparoscopy is a standard element of most investigations into a fertility problem. It is an invaluable test, providing information about the condition of the fallopian tubes which is vital to the assessment of a woman's reproductive capabilities.

You are told that you may expect pain in the shoulder after a laparoscopy, which is caused by left-over gas. It's a bit uncomfortable around the little incision, where you have a stitch or two, and you usually have a slightly sore stomach. The only other after-effect was what the doctor had described to me as a 'blue period', which is the dye coming out. I felt much more fragile after the laparoscopy than I had expected, and most people find they need to take a few days off work.

HYSTEROSALPINGOGRAM

This is another technique used to examine the fallopian tubes and uterus. A small tube is put through the cervix and a special dye injected through the tube into the womb. A number of X-rays are taken as the dye passes through, and any problems such as blockages or adhesions will show up.

This test is often described as being 'uncomfortable'. For some women it is a straightforward and relatively painless experience, but others find it very painful. It may be helpful to discuss the process with your doctor beforehand.

OTHER TESTS

The tests listed above are some of the basic examinations which are routinely carried out during infertility investigations before IVF is considered. There may be others, depending on individual circumstances. An endometrial biopsy is sometimes used to check progesterone production, and to make sure that ovulation is taking place. This involves taking a small sample of the womb lining a few days before a period is due and then examining it. It is a simple process and you don't usually have an anaesthetic.

Hysteroscopy is sometimes used to look at the womb. It can be carried out at the same time as a laparoscopy and involves putting a thin telescope through the cervix to check for any abnormalities in the womb. Fibroids, adhesions or any oddities in the shape of the womb would show up with this test.

It can take many months, even years, to get through the infertility tests. You may have a long wait to get an appointment to see a consultant in the first place, and as many of the tests can only be carried out at certain times of the month or have to be repeated it can become a lengthy process. In some cases the results will continue to be inconclusive.

OTHER TREATMENTS

Before you get to the stage of considering IVF you will often have had some other kind of treatment to try to help you conceive.

For women, drugs are often used to stimulate ovulation. It is important that you are monitored carefully during this treatment to check that the drugs are working, and a series of ultrasound scans is the best way to do this. Endometriosis may be treated with drugs or with surgery, although some doctors question the efficacy of these treatments in improving fertility. Tubal surgery may be carried out to repair damaged fallopian tubes, or fibroids may be surgically removed from the womb in an operation known as myomectomy.

Drug treatments are sometimes used for male fertility problems, and surgery may be suggested to clear the tubes which carry the sperm or to remove varicoceles, enlarged veins around the testicles which can affect sperm production. Often doctors will recommend going straight to assisted conception in these cases.

Intra-uterine insemination is a fairly simple form of assisted conception which is sometimes suggested. The man gives a sperm sample which is washed and then injected straight into the woman's womb at her most fertile time. Fertility drugs may be used during this treatment to try to improve the outcome.

HELPING YOURSELF

Sometimes more simple measures may make all the difference. Giving up smoking, losing weight or cutting down on drinking can have a considerable effect on your fertility and also improve your general health. Feeling that you are able to do something to improve your situation can help you to adopt a more positive attitude, and eating healthily and taking exercise may make you feel better about yourself, which can only be beneficial. However, it is equally important not to make yourself completely miserable by blaming yourself for your fertility problems just because you can't stand the thought of going to the gym or you ate chips for supper.

Recreational drug use is fairly widespread nowadays, but

should not form part of the lives of couples trying to conceive. Cannabis is often seen as a harmless and relaxing drug, but it can have a serious effect on sperm. Cutting it out may greatly improve your chances of a successful pregnancy.

IVF is more likely to work if you are generally healthy. Research has shown that IVF pregnancy rates are higher in couples who don't smoke cigarettes, and suggests that both eggs and sperm are affected by smoking. Women who are very overweight do not respond as well to the drugs given during IVF treatment.

WHEN CAN IVF HELP?

IVF means that fertilisation takes place outside the human body. The sperm and eggs are gathered and mixed together, usually in a small dish rather than in the test tube which has led to the concept of the test-tube baby. The aim is to get the sperm to fertilise the eggs to produce embryos. In order to maximise the chances of this happening, a woman is usually given drugs to stimulate her ovaries and to help them to produce lots of eggs, as not all of them will fertilise. If the process is successful, up to three embryos can be transferred back into the womb in the hope that one or more will implant and then develop.

When IVF was first used in the 1970s it was seen primarily as a way of treating women with blocked fallopian tubes, but it is now being used to treat a wide variety of female and male fertility problems. It is still most commonly considered when there are problems with the fallopian tubes as it offers a way of bypassing them by taking eggs from the ovary and replacing the fertilised embryos directly into the womb. It is often used when the female partner has endometriosis, and for male problems where there is a low sperm count or motility problems but the sperm are still capable of fertilising an egg. IVF can have a diagnostic value in cases of unexplained infertility, because it allows the whole fertilisation process to be carefully monitored and can shed light on the true nature of the fertility problem. It is important to be satisfied that unexplained infertility has been thoroughly investigated before embarking on such an expensive and invasive treatment, in case there is a more simple solution. Basic tests can be forgotten or ignored, especially if patients change clinics during investigations.

OTHER PROCEDURES

In some cases of male infertility a relatively new technique called ICSI, or intra-cytoplasmic sperm injection, may be suggested. ICSI involves injecting the sperm straight into the egg using a thin glass needle, rather than leaving the sperm to attempt to break through itself. Not all IVF clinics are licensed to perform ICSI, as embryologists have to be specially trained to carry out the procedure.

The use of ICSI has meant that many men with low sperm counts or motility, for whom IVF would not have worked, can now have a child of their own. Once, the only solution in such cases would have been to use donor sperm. There has been a huge increase in the demand for ICSI, and latest figures in the United Kingdom showed that the number of ICSI cycles had quadrupled in a year. The current success rates for this sort of treatment, known in general as micromanipulation, have also risen, and the live birth rate currently stands at around 19 per cent.

One new process which could help men with even more severe fertility problems involves using immature sperm, or spermatids, which are injected directly into the egg as in ICSI. This would allow men who do not produce mature sperm to father their own children. The technique has been used success-fully, and babies have been born using spermatids, but it is currently banned in the United Kingdom. Research projects are still going on, but the procedure is very new and it is felt that further investigations are needed to prove that it is completely safe before it can be used routinely.

GIFT, or gamete intra-fallopian transfer, is sometimes used

instead of IVF where there are no problems with the fallopian tubes. The eggs are collected in the same way, but instead of being fertilised in a dish they are just mixed with the sperm and then put back into the tubes. The advantage of GIFT is that fertilisation is able to take place in the natural environment of the woman's body, but the disadvantage is that if it doesn't work no information has been gained about whether the sperm ever succeeded in fertilising the eggs.

ZIFT, or zygote intra-fallopian transfer, is another variation. With ZIFT, the eggs are collected and mixed with the sperm. They are allowed to fertilise and are put back into the fallopian tubes two days later.

DONOR SPERM AND EGGS

Insemination by donor is widely used in cases of male infertility, and donor sperm can also be used in IVF treatment if there are problems with both partners, or to treat single women or lesbians. Using donor sperm is quite straightforward, but the implications are far-reaching for the child, its parents and the surrounding family. Special counselling is necessary to make sure that those opting for this route have thought through what they would tell their child if the treatment is successful, and have fully considered all the problems they may face in the future.

Donor eggs can be used if a woman isn't able to produce her own, and the use of a donated egg may enable a woman who has gone through a premature menopause to have a child through IVF. Success rates for IVF using donor eggs are higher than the routine IVF rates, partly due to the fact that women who wish to donate eggs must be relatively young. However, there are often long waiting lists for this treatment unless a woman has a female relative or friend who is willing to give eggs. Becoming a sperm donor is a relatively simple thing for a man to do and involves very little time, but a woman who donates her eggs needs a lot of commitment. She will have to undergo drug treatment and egg collection, neither of which are particularly pleasant experiences. It is one thing to go through the stimulation and retrieval process to try to create a much longed for child, but quite another to do it for purely altruistic reasons.

There are only about a thousand IVF cycles with donor eggs carried out in the whole of the United Kingdom each year, and a couple of hundred cycles with donated embryos. Most hospitals have far more women waiting for eggs than there are available donors. Egg-sharing schemes have been mooted as one way around this problem. Such schemes offer women who are having IVF a free treatment cycle if they agree to donate half the eggs they produce to other women who are waiting for a donor egg. Many doctors in the field are deeply concerned about such arrangements which they feel may cause more problems than they solve, particularly for the women who are donating the eggs. Egg-sharing schemes are not widely available.

There is an ongoing debate about the fact that children born of donor eggs or sperm have no legal right to find out who their parents are. The fact that a child was conceived using donor eggs or sperm is not mentioned on their birth certificate, and the donor is guaranteed anonymity by law. Many parents who use donors welcome this fact, and donors themselves would often not wish to be contacted. However, some critics claim the issue is currently dealt with too casually, and believe the children are being deprived of their rights. They feel that children born from donor eggs or sperm should have the same access to information about their background as those who have been adopted. In Sweden the law allows children access to their donor parents' identities, but this does not alter the fact that the donor bears no legal responsibility for a child conceived in this way. The issue is a moral minefield, and likely to remain the subject of much discussion.

Anyone who is considering using donor eggs or sperm should be given counselling, and it may be helpful to join the DI Network which provides help and advice for couples who are considering using donor gametes or who have done so. For women who need donor eggs there is a National Egg and Embryo Donation Society which may be useful, and an organisation called Daisy Chain which exists to help women who have gone through a premature menopause.

WHO IS ELIGIBLE FOR IVF?

Whether you will be eligible for IVF depends entirely on where you live, the clinic carrying out the treatment and whether you are paying for it. There is currently no national policy on the funding of fertility treatment in the United Kingdom, and the decision as to whether IVF is available under the auspices of the National Health Service depends entirely on where you live, as it is paid for by local health authorities. The majority of IVF cycles in the United Kingdom are funded privately, and many patients pay for their own treatment in NHS units.

Some local health authorities flatly refuse to pay for any assisted conception at all, whilst others will fund a limited number of IVF cycles for couples who fit certain set criteria. There may be an age limit for women, usually somewhere between thirty-five and forty, and the authority may say that couples must have been trying to conceive for a certain number of years. Many will only fund those who are childless, thus ruling out couples who have previously adopted or those with children from an earlier relationship along with those suffering from secondary infertility. There is almost always a limit on the number of cycles of treatment which will be funded, and sometimes only one will be paid for.

Clinics offering IVF have their own rules about who they are willing to treat, and many set age limits for women, usually somewhere between forty and fifty. Some will not treat women who are overweight.

Single Women and Lesbian Couples

Many clinics will only treat women who are in stable hetero-sexual relationships, and will not consider single women or lesbian couples. The Human Fertilisation and Embryology Act, which governs the way IVF is administered in the UK, states that 'a woman shall not be provided with treatment services unless account has been taken of the welfare of any child who may be born as a result of the treatment (including the need of that child for a father)'. This reference to the need for a father has sometimes been taken to mean that single women or lesbian couples should not be treated, but in fact the HFEA's Code of Practice states quite clearly that the Act does not intend to exclude any category of woman from being considered for treatment. Some clinics say they may be willing to treat a single woman or a woman in a lesbian relationship if their case is first referred to the hospital's ethics committee.

A single woman or one in a lesbian relationship who needs IVF to conceive may have to contact a number of clinics before finding one which is willing to offer treatment. Additionally, most local health authorities would not agree to fund IVF in these circumstances.

CHOOSING A CLINIC

All clinics which perform in vitro fertilisation in the United Kingdom have to be licensed by the Human Fertilisation and Embryology Authority before they start treating patients. The HFEA can provide an up-to-date list of units with details of the different types of treatment they are licensed to offer. In some areas there is a wide range of centres to choose from, all offering IVF at different prices, but in others there may only be one clinic unless you are willing to travel very long distances. Couples who hope to have their treatment funded by their local health authority will have to go to a clinic which the authority deals with, which usually means that there won't be a choice.

If your fertility investigations have been carried out in a clinic which offers IVF it will make sense to stay there unless you have strong reasons for moving. Tests often have to be repeated when patients change clinics, and the medical team will not have had a chance to familiarise themselves with your individual circumstances.

If you are in a position to decide where to have treatment, there are a number of factors which need to be taken into consideration.

Location

This is the most obvious factor. During the course of a treatment cycle it will be necessary to visit the clinic several times a week, and travelling long distances can add to the stress. What may seem a perfectly reasonable journey for an occasional appointment with a consultant may become unreasonable when it has to be done on a daily basis. Sometimes it is possible to have what is known as 'transport IVF', where most of the treatment is carried out at a local hospital and you only visit the IVF unit for crucial stages in the procedure. This kind of arrangement is becoming more common, but is only available at certain centres.

Cost of Treatment

This, too, is very important. The charges for IVF vary considerably, and paying more doesn't necessarily mean you will be more likely to have a successful outcome. It is often cheaper to pay for treatment as a private patient at a unit in an NHS hospital than to go to a private hospital. Individual clinics will send you their price lists on request, and the prices they quote are usually for one IVF cycle. This may not include charges for consultations, for any tests which have to be carried out beforehand, and for drugs. The drugs used in IVF are very expensive, and although it may be possible to get your GP to prescribe them, not all practitioners are willing to do so. If you have to pay for the drugs yourself it will add hundreds of pounds to the total bill.

One study in 1997 looked at the cost per live birth of IVF treatment at individual clinics. Using each unit's charges for a treatment cycle in conjunction with the individual success rates, researchers worked out how much on average a couple might spend to conceive a child there. Critics claimed that the figures were flawed because different items were included in the prices quoted by the various clinics and because the success rates depend so much on the type of patients treated. However, the figures, which ranged from £5,000 at best to over £40,000 at the other end of the scale, did reveal how costly IVF can be and how much the price may vary depending on where you are treated.

IVF is never cheap. For some couples, the cost means it simply isn't an option. This has led to accusations that it is a very discriminatory process which ultimately allows only the comfortably off the chance to try to have a child on this basis. Many couples spend tens of thousands of pounds and have to scrimp, save and borrow to afford their treatment. This may be fine when the treatment works, but can make it even more devastating when it doesn't.

Freezing Facilities

When drugs are used to stimulate the ovaries during an IVF cycle the aim is to produce a number of eggs which will then be mixed with the male partner's sperm in the hope that some of them will fertilise and produce embryos. Up to three embryos can be replaced in the woman's womb, but sometimes more will have been produced. Any spare embryos can be frozen and replaced at a later date in another cycle, provided the clinic you choose has freezing facilities. Some people, however, are not happy at the idea of using frozen embryos and prefer to let any spare ones perish or donate them to research. Clinics which do have facilities to freeze embryos often charge a one-off payment or an annual fee for storing them, and you will also have to pay when you have them replaced in your womb.

Waiting Times

These will differ from one clinic to another, and the time it takes
to get a first appointment to see a consultant, and for IVF itself,
should both be taken into consideration. If a woman cannot
produce eggs herself and will need to use donated eggs the
waiting time will probably be much longer, as there are never
enough donor eggs available to meet demand.

Success Rates

When making your choice of clinic this will probably be the
most deeply discussed factor. Before beginning to compare rates
it is essential to check exactly what figures are being given to
ensure that you are comparing like with like. Some clinics will
quote the pregnancy rate, which tells you the percentage of
women who have got pregnant after treatment; others use the
live birth rate, which is always lower because sadly some women
will miscarry in early pregnancy. You also need to check whether
the rates are being given for each treatment cycle, for each egg
collection or for each embryo transfer. Some IVF treatment
cycles have to be abandoned because of medical complications,
and not all will produce embryos, so the success rate for each
embryo transfer will be higher than the rate for each treatment
cycle.

Fortunately, there is now an easier way to compare success
rates. The Human Fertilisation and Embryology Authority pub-
lish their own figures, which show comparable rates at all the
clinics in the United Kingdom. They give the live birth rates for
each IVF treatment cycle – the 'take-home baby rate' – as well as
the success rates for donor insemination. Their figures have been
adjusted to take into consideration some of the factors which are
most likely to make a difference to a clinic's success rates: age of
patients, duration of infertility, any previously unsuccessful
treatments, previous pregnancies and poor sperm quality. This

is meant to give a comparable rate but even with these adjustments there is a fairly wide margin for error, especially in the figures for smaller clinics which may not carry out many IVF treatments.

Some consultants working in fertility units were very critical when the HFEA first published the success rates in 1995. It was felt that the figures could alarm patients, who would use the guide as a league table. The HFEA had stressed that the birth rates could vary greatly from one year to another, but when the information was published it was already nearly two years out of date.

It is important to remember the limitations of these figures and to take the other factors involved in choosing a clinic into consideration before making a choice. Large clinics which carry out more than two hundred IVF treatment cycles each year are generally more successful, with a live birth rate of around 16 per cent, while small clinics carrying out fewer than two hundred cycles have an average live birth rate of about 13 per cent. However, a small clinic may have other advantages, with staff who will get to know you personally and respond to your individual needs.

If you are in a position to choose a clinic, the most important thing is to find somewhere which you feel suits you, as IVF can be difficult and even traumatic at times. It is vital to feel happy with your choice of clinic before you embark on your first treatment cycle.

2

Starting a Treatment Cycle

When I was having my first IVF treatment cycle, an infuriating article appeared in a national newspaper which claimed that fertility clinics were witnessing an increasing number of patients who were choosing to have babies by IVF because they were too busy to have sex. Career couples were supposedly leading such hectic lives that they were far too exhausted to have intercourse – presuming they ever managed to find themselves at home at the same time – and were opting to spend thousands of pounds on a test-tube baby instead. Reading between the lines, there was no real evidence to back up these claims, but the article epitomised a certain attitude towards assisted conception: the idea that all you have to do is pay your money and nine months later you'll produce a child. The reality is that only 15 per cent of treatment cycles will result in the birth of a baby, and anyone who was too busy to have sex could not begin to find the time to have IVF.

It's a process which requires your total commitment during the treatment cycle, but that is something which anyone longing for a child of their own is only too happy to give. Once you start IVF, you may find it dominates every area of your life. I had expected the medical side of the treatment – the drugs, injections and scans – to be the most difficult part. In fact, those things can be surprisingly easy to handle and it is the emotional upheavals which may be unexpected and hard to cope with. I remember going to a press briefing on IVF long before I ever thought I'd get that far down the line of fertility treatment. An expert was explaining to a group of journalists that IVF wasn't an easy process for couples to go through. 'Can you imagine', he said, 'having to remember to sniff a drug every four hours throughout the day? That's what women going through IVF treatment have to do.' I often remembered those words during my first treatment cycle, because for me sniffing five times a day was one of the easiest things about it.

Once the decision has been made that IVF is the way ahead, and the practicalities of where to go for treatment and how to pay have been sorted out, the next stage is usually a discussion with the consultant or another member of the medical team to explain exactly what will be involved. Up until this point IVF has often seemed a last resort in the series of tests and treatments, a final stage which you may have been hoping you will never reach. The prospect can seem rather alarming as it becomes a reality.

I was quite surprised to find I had terrible qualms about interfering with nature as I approached my first treatment cycle. Suddenly I began to question whether it was right to meddle in this way, and whether not being able to have children was a way of life I should learn to accept as my destiny. There is something rather frightening and futuristic about the way we see IVF – the idea of human beings created in laboratories by scientists in white coats. In fact the miracles of the process remain firmly in the hands of nature, and the scientific procedures remain crude in comparison. IVF has more to do with creating the circumstances in which nature can go ahead and make babies than with creating babies itself.

COUNSELLING

At this stage you should be offered counselling. The Code of Practice set out by the Human Fertilisation and Embryology

Authority states that all clinics in the United Kingdom must offer their patients the opportunity to have counselling before they go ahead with IVF. It is recognised that going through the treatment process creates stress in most patients and that counselling can help, although there is no obligation to see a counsellor if you don't want to.

There are three types of counselling which may help during IVF treatment. The first is implications counselling, which the HFEA says must be made available to everyone. It deals with the implications of the treatment both for the couple and for any child born as a result. The second is support counselling, which offers emotional help at particularly stressful times before, during or after the treatment. The third type is therapeutic counselling, which deals with the wider consequences of infertility and of treatment. Therapeutic counselling may be provided by specialists outside the clinic itself.

Seeing a counsellor will give you a chance to air any concerns with someone impartial. Your consultant won't usually have time to discuss your emotional responses to IVF, but they are nevertheless a very important part of what you are going through. Talking to a counsellor should be seen not as indicating some kind of weakness, but as a normal part of helping to prepare yourself for your treatment.

Even if you decide initially that you don't want to see a counsellor, you can change your mind at any time during treatment. Sometimes free counselling is included in the price of your treatment, but at other places you will have to pay – find out before you start.

The most important thing is that you should feel happy with your counsellor. I didn't have any counselling during my treatment, but in retrospect I think I might have found it very helpful to see someone who specialised in dealing with fertility problems. I had been to see a general counsellor while I was on the waiting list for IVF, and found it a depressing experience. At that time I was upset and feeling that my partner and I were getting nowhere in spite of years of tests and treatments. I found myself in floods of tears sitting opposite a woman who kept saying, in what seemed to me a bored and unsympathetic voice, that it must be terrible not to be able to have children. She was more interested in discussing my family background, which didn't strike me as remotely relevant, and I didn't feel our meeting did me any good at all. If you go to a counsellor who is accustomed to dealing with infertility you aren't likely to have this kind of negative experience. There are some excellent counsellors around, but it is still important to feel sure you are seeing the right person for you as an individual.

SUPPORT GROUPS

Even if you decide you don't want counselling, it may be very helpful to join a support group. Many clinics offering IVF have patient support groups through which you can meet other people who are going through fertility treatment. If your unit doesn't have one there are two national groups in the United Kingdom, Issue and Child, which can offer advice and put you in touch with others. You have to pay to join these organisations, but the help they offer via their information sheets, magazines, telephone helplines and local groups can be invaluable.

Max and I had never liked the idea of support groups, but when someone set one up in our area we decided we should go along to see what it was like. We were agreeably surprised. For the first time ever we found ourselves in a roomful of people who were all going through the same thing, and who all understood what it was like not to be able to get pregnant and have a child. I felt an incredible sense of relief just to know that we weren't alone. So I wasn't the only person who shrivelled up inside when someone asked when we were going to get around to having children. That evening we were able to laugh together about some of the ridiculous things people had said and the ghastly experiences we'd had which had been so painful to go through alone. Max and I stayed in the group throughout our treatment and, although we didn't attend regularly, it was good to know we could go when we felt we needed it and that there were other people out there who understood.

Support groups can be useful sources of information about what is involved in treatment, about local clinics offering IVF or even complementary therapies. Some invite speakers who can discuss various aspects of treatment from an informed perspective, giving you the opportunity to ask questions you wouldn't have time for at the clinic.

TELLING OTHER PEOPLE

It can be difficult to decide whether to tell friends, family and colleagues you are going to have IVF. Your decision will depend on how open you are about your fertility problems in general. Some couples prefer to tell people and avoid having to answer awkward questions, whilst others can't face telling anyone at all.

The main problem about telling people you are trying IVF is that most of them won't understand much about it. They may assume that, because you are having treatment, you will inevitably get pregnant after the first cycle. Sometimes attempts to 'cheer you along' can make you feel even worse. People telling you that they are sure it is going to work can be quite hard to cope with when you know it is far more likely that it *won't* work the first time. On the other hand, if you don't tell other people you can't expect support or sympathy.

Max found it much easier to tell people we couldn't have children than I did. For a long time I didn't want anybody to know, but when we did tell people we were trying IVF they were excited for us, and interested in what was going on. In the early stages of the treatment cycle it was wonderful to have friends being so supportive, but by the time we were waiting to find out whether it had worked I didn't want to talk about it any more. I felt as if it wasn't just us privately waiting to find out whether it had been successful, but everyone we knew being fascinated by whether I'd had a period or not. I realised that, whatever happened, I wanted us to have time to absorb it ourselves first before we had to share it with all and sundry – but we weren't going to be given the time to do that.

Many people find that the best way to deal with the situation is to tell people that they are having IVF treatment, but only to tell their very closest friends and family when they are actually going through a treatment cycle. That way you don't have to share your day-to-day experiences with everyone, but people will be able to be sympathetic if and when you feel the need to share the details with them.

HIV TESTING

Some, but not all, clinics require patients to be screened for HIV before they have treatment. A straightforward blood test is all that is needed to tell whether a patient is HIV positive. If your unit insists you have this test you should be offered counselling.

The IVF treatment of patients who are HIV positive is a controversial area. Some doctors feel that because such patients are at risk of developing AIDS and could pass the virus on to a baby during pregnancy or birth it would be wrong to help them conceive. Others argue that couples who risk passing on genetic diseases to their children are often treated, and that patients with HIV should not be regarded any differently.

There are no national regulations on the subject, and the decision on whether or not to treat a couple if one or both potential parents are HIV positive lies entirely with the treatment centre. The Human Fertilisation and Embryology Authority Code of Practice simply says that clinics should consider the welfare of any potential child and the health of the couple who want treatment. It is likely that a decision on an individual case would have to be considered by the local ethics committee, and ultimately it may be difficult to find a clinic willing to treat a patient who is HIV positive.

CONSENT FORMS

In the United Kingdom, you will have to sign a consent form from the Human Fertilisation and Embryology Authority before you can start a treatment cycle. There are two forms, one for men and one for women. Even for those who are not having treatment in the UK, the issues they address are worth considering before you start IVF.

The first part of the form deals with the use of eggs and sperm. In it you give consent for your eggs or sperm to be used to treat yourself and your partner. You may also give consent here for any spare eggs or sperm to be used to treat others, or to be donated to research projects. Many hospitals need donated eggs or sperm for specific research programmes. In this situation the staff should explain exactly what the research involves, and what would be done with your eggs or sperm. It is entirely up to you whether you donate any spare eggs or sperm, and you should never feel pressurised to agree to anything. It is not currently possible to freeze eggs.

The second half of the consent form deals with the storage of sperm and embryos. The law allows embryos to be frozen and stored for up to ten years. This will only apply if you produce more embryos than you can use in one treatment cycle, which is not always the case. Although the use of frozen embryos has become widespread, some people have concerns about freezing and do not wish to keep spare embryos in this way. It is not currently possible to freeze eggs.

You are also asked to consider what should be done with embryos, and with sperm for the male partner, if you should die or become mentally incapacitated. You can ask for them to be allowed to perish, or to continue to be kept in storage and used to treat your partner, to treat others or to be used for research.

The need for written consent in such cases was highlighted in the United Kingdom by the case of Diane Blood, who wanted to use sperm from her late husband to try to have a child. He had not given written consent for this before he died, and she had a long legal battle in order to get permission to use his sperm for artificial insemination abroad.

It can seem daunting to have to consider such weighty issues before you have even started the treatment process, but it is important to think through your decisions carefully. The process of creating embryos in vitro is strictly regulated, and the consent forms are intended to ensure you have complete control over what happens to the embryos you are hoping to make. Once all this has been sorted out, you will be able to arrange a date to start your treatment cycle at your clinic.

DRUGS

The drugs you take during your IVF cycle will be slightly different at every treatment centre. Each clinic has its own drug regime which will be adapted to suit you. The aim remains the same: to get the ovaries to produce a number of eggs which will then be collected.

If you are going to ask your GP to prescribe the drugs for you the clinic will write a letter listing what you need. Some GPs are happy to do this, others are not. You should find out your own GP's policy as soon as you can, as these drugs are extremely expensive to buy yourself. If your GP will not prescribe them, some hospitals will sell you the drugs from their own pharmacy – this can be cheaper than buying them from a private pharmacist. Check the relative prices before deciding what to do; the medical team treating you should be able to offer advice.

If in the end you have to obtain your drugs through an ordinary pharmacy, take your prescription along well before you start your treatment. Although IVF is becoming more common, most local chemists won't keep stocks of such expensive drugs on hand just in case someone might want them. They usually have to be ordered, which can take several days. There have been shortages of some of the drugs, and this can sometimes lead a pharmacist to suggest replacing one of those on your list with a similar drug when the exact one is not available. If your pharmacist is experiencing any sort of difficulty ask for advice at your clinic. The staff will be able to tell you whether they would be happy with a substitute, or give you details of where you might be able to get the specific drugs prescribed.

Suppressing the Ovaries

Most treatment cycles will begin with the use of a drug to suppress your natural cycle and thus make your ovaries more receptive to the stimulating drugs which follow. These suppressants are products such as Buserelin or Goserelin, which are usually taken either as a nasal spray at regular intervals throughout the day, by injection twice daily or by implant. If you have the spray you will have to remember to use it every four hours, which some women find awkward, but it may be preferable if you don't like injections.

Exactly when you start taking the suppressing drug will depend on the regime used at your clinic. Sometimes you will start taking it towards the end of your cycle, and then start the drugs to stimulate the ovaries in the next cycle, or you may start both at the same time. Usually you will continue to take this drug until you have your final injection before egg collection.

I was due to start sniffing in the middle of a week away filming in Scotland, and I was quite worried about being so far from home in case something ghastly happened. I'd been told that the nasal spray could cause menopausal side-effects (see below), but I had no idea how long they might take to develop or how serious they might be. I remember feeling terribly lonely as I sat in my hotel bedroom on the morning of the first sniffing day, waiting for the clock to reach seven, the appointed hour for the first sniff.

In fact, nothing happened at all and it was rather an anticlimax. The only thing you are likely to notice straightaway if you use a nasal spray is a rather horrid taste at the back of your throat. It is quite difficult to remember to sniff at exactly the right time to keep the doses spaced out evenly throughout the day, especially if you are busy. Some women find it helpful to use an alarm clock or watch to remind themselves when to sniff. It may sound strange, but I quite enjoyed having to remember to sniff. It helped me to think I was finally on my way to doing something about not being able to get pregnant.

Side-effects

The suppressing drug produces an artificial menopause, and some women find they have side-effects such as headaches, mood changes or hot flushes which are common in menopausal women. Also, the spray can irritate your nostrils if you are using it for a prolonged period of time.

Stimulating the Ovaries

The next drug taken will make the ovaries produce more eggs than usual. In a woman's natural cycle, a number of follicles will start growing each month but only one will become dominant and go on to produce an egg. This part of the IVF treatment cycle aims to get more follicles to carry on growing in the hope that there will be more eggs.

A number of different types of drugs are given. The first generation of drugs which may be used are products derived from human menopausal urine, such as Pergonal or Humegon. The second are slightly purer forms of these drugs, such as Metrodin HP, and the third generation are very pure drugs such as Gonal-F and Puregon, which contain no other substances. These newer, purer drugs are much more expensive, and many clinics would rather use the older, cheaper drugs and keep costs down because they don't believe there is really any difference in the effect on the ovaries.

There are various different brands of these drugs, and the amount each individual takes will be adjusted to meet what the medical team feel will be most suitable for you. If you have been taking a suppressing drug you will continue to do so all the time you are having these stimulating drugs, as this allows the medical team to have greater control over your cycle.

The story you will probably hear at some stage about these

stimulating drugs is that they are made from nuns' urine – which in fact isn't quite as crazy as it may sound. The hormones in these drugs are produced by women at the time of the menopause. As their ovaries stop working, women's bodies produce more and more of these hormones in an attempt to restart them. The excess hormones leave the body in the urine. In the 1960s a way of extracting the hormones from the urine was discovered, but huge quantities of urine were needed to obtain a small quantity of hormones. The drug was developed in Italy, where researchers needed to find lots of post-menopausal women to donate urine, and the most obvious place to look was in convents. Some of the drugs are still made using this process, although the urine is collected from many older women and not exclusively from nuns.

Injections

These stimulating drugs are given by daily injection, and you or your partner may want to try to do it yourselves. Although this may sound unpleasant at first, it's worth giving it a go as it makes things so much easier. If you don't, you will have to go to the clinic every day, or find a friendly local doctor or nurse to do it for you. There are self-injector kits available which make the process less daunting: once you have prepared the syringe all you have to do is load it into a plastic device, hold it against the skin and press the trigger. As this is an intra-muscular injection given in the thigh or the buttock, it's not difficult to get it right.

I'm quite squeamish about injections and couldn't face the idea of doing it myself, but Max was quite keen to try as it meant he could be more involved in the process which was otherwise entirely focussed on me. It all seemed far more complicated than we'd imagined, because we had to mix the solution ourselves before we could get down to any actual injecting. There were little glass ampoules of saline solution, and others containing a white powder in a small ball at the bottom of the ampoule. The dates on each ampoule had to be checked first, and the glass tops broken off. Then the ampoules of powder had to be mixed with the saline to dissolve them, which was done by drawing the saline into the syringe and shooting it out into the ampoule of powder. It seemed a rather serious business, and made us feel like chemists in a laboratory as we mixed up our daily potion.

After all that, the injecting part seemed fairly straightforward. We got detailed instructions and a bit of stabbing practice at the unit, jabbing the needle into the fruit the sister had brought for her lunch. Doing the first injection at home alone was a bit unnerving, but once we had done it we were rather proud of ourselves and to my surprise I didn't feel it at all.

Side-effects

The drugs which stimulate your ovaries often make your abdomen feel bloated as the follicles grow larger, and it can be quite uncomfortable. I remember saying I felt like an over-ripe fruit towards the end of the injections. They can cause mood swings, aching muscles and joints, and allergic reactions around the place where the needle has been injected. However, many women experience no side-effects at all.

I always felt quite distracted, absent-minded and vague during treatment, and had assumed this was some kind of side-effect from the drugs. I was surprised to find I felt exactly the same when I did a frozen embryo cycle without any drugs, and I realised my supposed side-effects had more to do with the emotional stress of the treatment than with the drugs. I was quite surprised that the stress alone had such a noticeable effect, as I had thought I was feeling relatively together at the time. IVF is a very intense emotional experience, and you shouldn't underestimate the way this can affect you.

MONITORING YOUR TREATMENT

Throughout this stage of treatment the medical team will be monitoring the development of the growing follicles very closely. This involves regular ultrasound scans, usually through the insertion of a probe into the vagina. You will be able to see the follicles growing, although you will probably need to have the scan picture explained to you. There may be blood tests throughout this time to check your hormone levels, which should increase as the follicles grow. The levels of the drugs you are taking may be adjusted, depending on how the follicles are growing.

About 80 per cent of women respond well to the drugs, but some treatment cycles have to be cancelled because women either over-respond to the drugs (see Ovarian Hyperstimulation Syndrome below), or don't respond at all. If a treatment cycle has to be cancelled or delayed it is important not to get too despondent, as getting the right dose of drugs for an individual can take some working out.

Ovarian Hyperstimulation Syndrome

One thing the medical team will be watching for as they monitor the development of the follicles is the threat of ovarian hyper-stimulation syndrome, which occurs when the drugs cause the ovaries to produce too many follicles. It can lead to swelling of the ovaries and fluid collecting in the abdomen and around the lungs. If there is a serious risk of ovarian hyperstimulation syndrome, the clinic will stop the treatment cycle immediately. Usually the condition can be treated by resting in bed and drinking lots of fluid, and it will cause only mild pain. It can become more serious in a small percentage of women who will have to be treated in hospital. Women who suffer from poly-cystic ovary syndrome are more at risk of hyperstimulation, and will be monitored more closely.

BALANCING TREATMENT AND WORK

You will probably be going to the clinic three or four times a week at this stage and it can be quite stressful. Nevertheless many women are glad to be at work during this part of their treatment because it keeps their minds occupied with other things. If you can arrange for all your scans and blood tests to be done at a time which suits you, it may be possible to continue working without too much disruption. Some clinics do the scans and blood tests very early in the morning so you can fit them in before work.

I tried working through the treatment cycle the first time, and found it was impossible. I hadn't told anyone what I was doing, but I'd said I had a lot of hospital appointments and wouldn't be able to travel away from home for a couple of weeks. I was asked to go to Northern Ireland for a week as soon as the treatment cycle started, which I managed to explain would be impossible, but then I had to keep fending off early starts miles away from home on days I was meant to be going to the clinic. In the end I was more worried about how I could cope with working and going to the clinic than I was about the treatment cycle itself, and I took a week's leave to restore my sanity and get me through the rest of the cycle. The next time I told my boss in advance and took ten days off from the start of the injections, which I found made it much easier to cope.

A lot depends on the job you do and how straightforward it is for you to fit visits to the clinic around your work. It may also depend on whether you have told your colleagues about your treatment. If you can tell your immediate superior you won't need to invent plausible reasons for being late for work three times a week, but if you don't have a good working relationship that may be out of the question. I was lucky to be working for a very sympathetic boss who was extremely understanding, but when the first treatment cycle didn't work I was quite glad I hadn't told anyone else. That would have meant I had to cope with colleagues offering their commiserations, which can be surprisingly hard to handle.

MATURING THE EGGS

The follicles are measured carefully by ultrasound, and when enough have reached a satisfactory size you are ready to go on to the next stage. The eggs have to ripen before they are ready to be collected, and an injection of hCG – human chorionic gonado-trophin, such as Pregnyl or Profasi – is needed to help them mature. The timing of this injection is very important as the eggs have to be at exactly the right stage when they are collected. It is normally done very late at night, and once it has been given you will stop taking your suppressing drug. After this last injection you will have a day with no drugs at all while the eggs are ripening. They are collected about thirty-five hours after the injection.

The hCG injection is the final part of this stage of treatment. The ovaries have been stimulated and should have produced eggs. You can now proceed to the next part of the treatment cycle, in which the in vitro fertilisation itself will occur – taking the eggs out of the body and fertilising them before replacing them in the womb.

3

Eggs and Embryos

From the moment Max and I started our first IVF treatment, egg collection had seemed to me the focal point of
the whole process. I imagined that once we arrived at that
stage we would be on our way to the home straight, and I felt
quite exhilarated when we reached egg collection day.

Most clinics do egg collections in the morning, and you may
have to get there quite early. The man will be asked to produce a
semen sample on arrival. It can be difficult to have to perform to
order like this, especially at such a crucial stage of the treatment
cycle. You shouldn't feel embarrassed if you think you might
have problems, but if you are worried about it do let the staff at
the clinic know in advance – it will make you even more stressed
on the day if you haven't discussed your concerns beforehand. If
you live close to the clinic, you may be able to produce a sample
at home and bring it in with you. Alternatively, consider freezing
some sperm in advance which can be used on the day as back-up.

Once the man has given a sample it is taken to the laboratory
where an embryologist examines it and checks that the sperm
count is satisfactory. The team will have advised you how long to
abstain from intercourse before the day in order to get the best
possible sample. You may be asked for a second sample if the
count is low. The embryologist separates the sperm from the

surrounding seminal fluid, and keeps the sperm ready to be put with the eggs once they have been collected.

Egg collection is quite a delicate process, during which women are either put under general anaesthetic or heavily sedated. Ultrasound is usually used to identify the ovaries and follicles, and then a fine needle is inserted into each of the follicles and the fluid they contain is sucked out. If there is an egg inside the follicle it will be sucked out along with the fluid, but not all follicles contain eggs. The embryologist checks the fluid for eggs as it is flushed out.

Sometimes egg collection is done by laparoscopy. A small incision is made by the naval and a laparoscope, which is used to look at the ovaries and follicles, is inserted along with the needle to empty out the follicles. If a laparoscopy is involved you will need a general anaesthetic, but the procedure is in any case rare nowadays.

I was rather looking forward to egg collection, until the moment we arrived at the clinic bright and early one morning. I'd read everything I could find about IVF and I knew what was going to happen, but I had somehow persisted in clinging to a mental vision of egg collection as a slightly glorified smear test. When the doctor and nurse changed into operating theatre garments and began to talk about the imminent procedure as 'the operation' I felt terrified.

One of the advantages of having the egg collection done by ultrasound under sedation is that your partner can usually be with you throughout the whole process. I found it very reassuring, as Max was allowed to sit right next to me which made it feel less like an operation. Once I was in my hospital gown lying on the table, the doctor put a needle into the back of my hand which she explained was for the sedatives. As soon as I'd had them everything started to seem distant and strange, as if I was watching what was going on in a half-asleep state from just outside my body.

Doctors often describe egg collection as 'uncomfortable', but most women who have been through the procedure say it hurts. Although the drugs make you feel very hazy, you may still feel pain at times, but it isn't a constant pain and I found it bearable. When the needle was put into the follicle and the egg sucked out, it felt a bit like having a tooth drilled without any anaesthetic. The rest of the time it didn't hurt at all. Max found it quite upsetting to watch the first time we had the eggs collected, as it was obviously hurting me, but the second time was a lot easier as he knew what to expect. Women who have had a number of IVF treatment cycles often find that each egg collection feels different; sometimes it can be extremely painful, whilst other collections are quite easy. Some prefer to have the egg collection done under general anaesthetic.

The fluid which is sucked out of the follicle goes down a tube and is then examined by the embryologist. I was aware of her calling out each time she found an egg. Once all the follicles have been emptied, the embryologist tells everyone how many eggs have been collected. The number can vary considerably, but in an average cycle will probably be around nine or ten. Very occasionally there will be no eggs at all. If this happens you will need to discuss with the medical team why this might have happened, and decide what you should do next.

When the operation is over you will have to rest at the unit for a while until the staff are happy that you are well enough to leave. It is usually possible to go home within a few hours, but you will probably feel extremely tired and you must not drive or operate any kind of machinery for the rest of the day.

FERTILISATION

Once the eggs have been collected, the embryologist gets to work. The eggs and sperm are mixed together in a special culture in a dish, and left overnight in an incubator to allow fertilisation to take place. I'd been so obsessed with the idea of the eggs being collected that it hadn't crossed my mind to worry about whether they would fertilise. I was surprised to find I felt very nervous about it. It was all very well having produced a number of eggs, but if none of them fertilised that would be the end of the cycle.

That's what makes IVF such a difficult experience: as soon as you are congratulating yourself at having got over one hurdle, you find yourself face to face with the next one. It was odd lying in bed that night to think of our eggs and sperm lying in a dish in a darkened laboratory. It seemed so far away from the way nature intended reproduction to take place, with the fertilisation process going on inside my body.

The embryologist checks the eggs to see if they have fertilised, which usually happens within twenty-four hours. On average about three-quarters of the eggs fertilise, but in up to 10 per cent of cases none of them will – due to the condition of the eggs or of the sperm, or an incompatibility problem. If none of your eggs fertilises, the consultant should discuss the possible reasons with you, and help you to decide what you should consider next.

Eggs that have fertilised are kept in the laboratory where they develop to form an embryo. The embryo divides into two separate cells, and will continue to divide over the following days. Embryos are usually replaced in the womb two or three days after egg collection. The embryologist assesses the quality of the embryos and grades them so that the best ones can be selected.

THE RISK OF A MULTIPLE BIRTH

Multiple births were once a rarity, but the advent of fertility drugs has led to a boom in twins and triplets. In 1995 there were nearly ten thousand sets of twins born in the United Kingdom, and around three hundred sets of triplets. The number of sets of triplets born increased three-fold between 1985 and 1995. The risk of a multiple birth is something you must consider seriously if you are taking any drug to boost your fertility. As in vitro fertilisation techniques have become more successful, so the multiple birth rate for IVF babies has increased to reach an alarming 32 per cent.

The risks of multiple births were highlighted in the United Kingdom by the case of Mandy Allwood, a woman who became pregnant with eight babies and later miscarried, losing them all. She had not been having IVF treatment, but had been taking some of the drugs which are often used in IVF cycles. The case drew attention to the general lack of knowledge and confusion about fertility treatment, as it was often presumed that she had had IVF and she was even referred to by some newspapers as the woman who had 'lost octuplets produced by IVF treatment'. Her story led to calls for fertility drugs to be more strictly regulated, as such a pregnancy should be virtually impossible if the drugs are used responsibly. Exactly what went wrong in Mandy Allwood's case has never been clear, although it seems she had unprotected intercourse after taking part of a course of drugs which had already successfully stimulated her ovaries to produce a number of eggs. Normally a woman taking these drugs would be closely monitored, and if a large number of follicles were seen to be developing she would be warned that she must under no circumstances have unprotected intercourse. Many consultants have long been concerned that, while procedures like IVF which involve creating embryos outside the body are monitored rigorously, the use of fertility drugs alone is not.

The law in the United Kingdom would not allow such a multiple pregnancy to occur as a result of IVF treatment. If there are a number of embryos, more than one is usually replaced to increase the chances of pregnancy, but no more than three may be put back. More and more clinics are now recommending that couples have just two embryos replaced, particularly if the woman is under thirty-five, it is her first IVF attempt and the embryos are of good quality.

When you have been trying to get pregnant for years, the prospect of a multiple birth can seem an instant solution and it is easy to imagine the joys of a ready-made family. However, there are serious risks involved even with a triplet pregnancy. Not only is the miscarriage rate much higher, but there is also a greater risk of complications throughout pregnancy and in labour, of premature birth, low birth weight, disability and neonatal death. The average length of a triplet pregnancy is thirty-five weeks compared to an average of forty weeks for a singleton pregnancy, and the average birth weight of a triplet is just 4 lb compared to an average of 7 lb 5 oz for a single baby. Inevitably, babies born so much earlier and weighing so much less are more vulnerable and more likely to suffer problems in their early days.

It is worth noting that data from the Human Fertilisation and Embryology Authority shows that, when more than four embryos have been created, the live birth rate is 23.4 per cent when just two embryos are put back. Putting three embryos back in such cases makes surprisingly little difference, with a live birth rate of 24.4 per cent. The reasons for this are being investigated. It may be partly explained by the fact that couples who make the decision to have two embryos replaced rather than three are more likely to be those who have a good prognosis in the first place. However, the risks involved in a triplet pregnancy may make it worth considering having just two embryos replaced even when more are available.

FROZEN EMBRYOS

If a number of embryos have been produced it is often possible to freeze any spare ones and store them in liquid nitrogen. They can be thawed and used later in a natural cycle without going through the process of stimulating the ovaries with drugs and collecting the eggs (see also Frozen Embryo Cycles below).

There are, however, some drawbacks. Up to a third of embryos will not survive the freezing and thawing process. Even if they do survive, frozen embryos are less likely to implant than fresh embryos: only about 11 per cent of frozen embryo transfers end in a live birth. It is quite possible to have a number of embryos frozen and for none of them to get through the thawing process. Some couples consider their frozen embryos as frozen babies, and it can be very difficult to cope if they do not survive to be replaced in the womb.

Not everyone is happy with the idea of using frozen embryos. There have been suggestions that the process should only be used when it would not be possible to use fresh embryos, and that there may be long-term effects as yet unknown. However, freezing is carried out routinely in IVF clinics and most consultants are perfectly happy that it is safe. Although critics claim it is a relatively new procedure, the first child from a frozen embryo was born in 1984, just six years after the first IVF baby. The most recent figures show that each year there are about five thousand frozen embryo transfers in the United Kingdom, and just under six hundred babies are born as a result. The Human Fertilisation and Embryology Authority has investigated the use of frozen embryos and found no evidence that freezing is harmful for patients or their potential children, but did add that there was a need for more follow-up studies. Research into possible risks is continuing.

It is possible to keep frozen embryos in storage for up to ten years in the United Kingdom. In 1990 the time limit had been set at five years, but there was a great outcry in 1995 when thousands of embryos reached the five-year limit, and the rules were changed to allow them to be stored for ten years if patients gave their 'written and informed consent'. Clinics faced the difficult task of tracing thousands of former patients, and by the time the deadline arrived 3,300 embryos had to be destroyed because the patients hadn't been found, or hadn't replied to letters from their doctors. A candlelit vigil was held outside Westminster Cathedral for the 'orphan' embryos, anti-abortion groups called for childless couples to be allowed to 'adopt' them, and an Italian research foundation offered to buy them. There were claims that the ultimate destruction of more than three thousand embryos was tantamount to infanticide, and the episode brought IVF a lot of adverse publicity as it was felt this had marked an alarming change in society's attitude to human life.

Frozen Embryo Cycles

As frozen embryos can usually be transferred in a natural cycle, there is no need to take all the drugs to stimulate the ovaries or to go through the egg collection process. But for women who have irregular cycles, who do not ovulate or who are using donated embryos, it may be necessary to use drugs. Even when a woman is having a frozen embryo transfer in a natural cycle, she will still have to make regular visits to the clinic. The medical team have to monitor her cycle very closely with regular ultrasound scans and blood tests to make sure the embryos are replaced at the best time, which is shortly after ovulation. The embryo transfer is exactly the same as in a normal IVF cycle.

EGG FREEZING

Ripe eggs are very fragile and therefore much more difficult to freeze than embryos or sperm. Although the process has been carried out successfully and a child has been born from a frozen egg, it is generally considered much too dangerous to carry out on a routine basis as there is a high risk of damage to the chromosomes, which could lead to genetic disease. However, there is a lot of research going on in this area and it is hoped that it will be possible to freeze eggs rather than embryos at some stage in the future. This would be a huge step forward.

EMBRYO TRANSFER

The embryo transfer itself is a fairly straightforward procedure which feels a bit like a smear test and takes only a matter of minutes. It may be possible to see your embryos before they are replaced. In some clinics this is done as a routine matter, but in others it is not offered at all. When we got to the hospital for our first embryo transfer, the embryologist asked us if we'd like to go and see our embryos. It felt extraordinary to see what might one day be our child when it consisted only of a few minuscule cells. In the laboratory we looked through a microscope at a little dish of liquid containing the three tiny blobs which were about to be put inside me. It seemed impossible that they would ever be able to grow into a person.

The woman's partner should be able to be with her for the embryo transfer. The embryologist will have selected the best of the embryos, and the prospective parents, with the advice of the medical team, will have decided how many are going to be replaced. The embryos are drawn up from the dish into a catheter, which is a thin, flexible plastic tube. The woman lies down and a speculum is put into her vagina to enable the doctor carrying out the transfer to see the cervix, or neck of the womb. The catheter is then passed through the cervix into the womb and the embryos are transferred. The doctor removes the catheter and passes it back to the embryologist, who examines it to make sure that all the embryos have gone. Sometimes the transfer is monitored by ultrasound to allow a further visual check that the embryos have gone back into the right place. The embryo transfer can be a bit uncomfortable, but it isn't a painful process. Once the embryos have been transferred the woman usually lies still for a while before leaving the clinic.

It's a very strange feeling, knowing that the precious embryos you have spent so long creating are now in your womb. I felt terrified to stand up after they'd been replaced in case they fell straight out again, and it's quite a common reaction. In fact you can carry on as normal as soon as they have been transferred. Some clinics will prescribe the hormone progesterone in pessaries or injections for the next two weeks, which is meant to help prepare the lining of the womb to encourage the embryos to implant.

Some women are elated after having their embryos transferred, feeling that they have reached the high point of the treatment cycle. Others find that they are unexpectedly anxious and frightened. On the way home from the hospital after our first embryo transfer I was suddenly overwhelmed by gloom and burst into tears. After all the weeks of being carefully monitored and looked after I felt so alone. No one could do anything more to help me, and I was so sure that I was incapable of having a child and of protecting the embryos which had been put inside me. I kept thinking of the tiny blobs we'd seen under the microscope. They seemed so absurdly small and vulnerable that I was sure my body, which had so far failed miserably to get pregnant, would not be up to nurturing them and helping them grow.

WAITING

The two weeks of waiting is by far the most difficult stage of an IVF cycle. Before you start, you imagine that once you have got through the drugs and the clinical procedures things will be easy. It came as a surprise to me that the hard part would be the time when nothing happens at all.

It is very common to worry about what you can and cannot do during this two-week waiting period. There is really very little you can do to affect the outcome, but it does make sense to try to be as healthy as possible. I was told not to drink any alcohol at all, and if you do drink during this time you should strictly limit your intake. The same goes for smoking. You may be told not to have intercourse. This is not because of any clear evidence that intercourse has an adverse effect at this stage, but more to stop you blaming yourselves for a possibly unsuccessful outcome if you have sex during the waiting period. You are often advised to avoid any strenuous activity, and it is easy to worry about what exactly constitutes 'strenuous'. However, it is most unlikely that you would do anything in your normal day-to-day activities which would threaten your chances of success.

If you have a job, you may be told to consider taking a few days off to rest afterwards. Some people like to be at home at this time, but I always found it useful to go back to work as soon as I could manage. It was really difficult to think about anything apart from whether the treatment had been successful or not, and I found that being at work was the only way to keep my mind occupied with other things for at least some of the time. I always used to think that the ideal solution would be to go to sleep for a fortnight and wake up in time for the outcome.

If you have decided to tell your friends and relatives that you are going through an IVF cycle they may start to drive you quite insane during these two weeks. A lot of people assume that IVF will inevitably work because you have paid such a lot of money, spent so long waiting and gone through so much. They may insist on treating you as if you are pregnant: 'Well, you are at the moment, aren't you, because you've got those embryos inside you,' they say. They probably imagine they are offering encouragement, but it can be very difficult to handle; whilst part of you may rejoice in finally being treated as a pregnant woman, another more cynical part is already angry with yourself for colluding with the pretence.

However well meant their enquiries may be, after years of dealing with not being pregnant by yourself it can be very hard to have to share the moment with all your friends and relatives. You can feel the eager anticipation in people's voices when they ask if there is 'any news' yet. I found it horribly intrusive. It made me feel my body was no longer my own in a way that even the treatment hadn't managed, as I knew that everyone was waiting to hear whether my period had arrived or not. The worst thing is that you end up feeling cross and angry with yourself for getting so fed up with people who are only trying to be sympathetic. Whatever anyone says to you at this stage is likely to seem wrong in some way or another and you just have to accept that it is going to be difficult to deal with people who know you are waiting.

Max wished we hadn't told anyone, because he got so annoyed by people asking whether the treatment had worked. The constant questions made him feel very tense and he couldn't concentrate on anything else at all. After going through it twice we told very few people the third time around, which made the whole process much easier to deal with.

When you're so experienced at not being pregnant, you will have become incredibly well versed in the symptoms of early pregnancy and are likely to find yourself constantly checking for the slightest sign. You may feel horribly aware of your body, and every little twinge or ache becomes magnified as you focus on it and try to analyse it. You peer down at your stomach as you pull on your jeans and wonder whether it appears slightly more rounded than usual. You feel a wave of nausea on the bus on your way to work and convince yourself for thirty blissfully happy seconds that you *must* be pregnant. Your body feels tender and you do feel terribly tired. Then you realise that the tiredness is probably due to the night you spent tossing and turning in bed wondering whether the treatment has worked, that the tenderness might just as easily be a premenstrual symptom and that the nausea is probably the result of the lurching and jolting of the bus as it makes its halting progress through the jammed commuter traffic. You pick up a heavy bag of shopping in the supermarket on the way home, feel your stomach muscles contract and are suddenly convinced that you have caused a miscarriage, which means you spend the evening in a state of depression convinced that it is entirely your fault that you won't be pregnant.

Your mind goes round and round in circles. You don't dare hope that you might be pregnant, but then you start to worry that if you don't believe it might have worked your negativity might make it fail.

Nothing is going to make this stage any easier, and nothing you can do will make the treatment more likely to succeed. You just have to accept that it is going to be a horrible fortnight and try to be as kind to yourselves as you can. If you can manage to relax and do things you both enjoy, to eat healthily and not to worry any more than is possible, you will be doing extremely well.

4

When Treatment Doesn't Work

After all the emotional highs and lows of the treatment cycle and the two-week wait, most couples are feeling incredibly tense when the moment finally arrives to discover whether their treatment cycle has worked. Some women will realise the cycle hasn't worked before the two weeks are up, as their period will start early. For others a pregnancy test will be necessary.

PREGNANCY TESTING

Some, but not all, clinics will arrange for you to have a pregnancy test two weeks after the embryo transfer. This will usually be a blood test: if an embryo has implanted and started to grow, it produces a hormone called human chorionic gonadotrophin which can be detected very easily in the blood.

Other clinics will ask you to do a pregnancy test yourself at home. The pregnancy hormone can also be detected in the urine, and a home test will involve checking a urine sample. You can buy a wide variety of home pregnancy testing kits in chemists and supermarkets. Most are very straightforward to use and come with clear instructions, though they are all slightly different and some are more sensitive than others. Some have to be done first thing in the morning with a urine sample produced as soon as you get out of bed because it will be more concentrated, whilst others can be done at any time of day. It is worth asking the medical staff at your clinic if they can recommend a home test kit if you are not sure which one to buy.

Home testing is quite accurate, but false negative tests in very early pregnancy are not uncommon, which is why a lot of the kits on sale contain two separate tests. You are advised to do the second test if an early result was negative but your period does not arrive. It is also possible to get a false positive if you have been having injections which contain the pregnancy hormone, but your clinic will be able to tell you whether a home test would be accurate in your case, and to advise you if you are unsure about the result.

With blood tests, which are highly sensitive, it is possible to have a 'low positive' result. This means that, although pregnancy hormones have been detected, the body is not producing them at a level which would normally suggest a successful implantation. Sometimes this means the pregnancy will not continue, and a period will follow within the next few days. It can also indicate an ectopic pregnancy. If you have a low positive result and it isn't followed by a period, you will have to return to the clinic for more blood tests or scans to make sure the levels of the pregnancy hormone are rising and that the embryo is developing.

ECTOPIC PREGNANCY

In an ectopic pregnancy the embryo implants outside the womb, usually in the fallopian tube. The pregnancy will not be able to survive as there is no room for the embryo to develop or for its support system, the placenta, to grow normally. Blood tests and ultrasound scans allow ectopic pregnancies to be detected early, which is important, because if the embryo keeps growing it can cause internal bleeding and may rupture the fallopian tube. Surgery is necessary as soon as an ectopic pregnancy is detected, but new techniques mean the tube can sometimes be saved by removing the pregnancy through laparoscopy or by injecting a drug which causes it to be reabsorbed into the body.

Although the embryo will have been inserted into the womb rather than into the fallopian tube during IVF, it is still possible to have an ectopic pregnancy as embryos can move about after they have been transferred. Women who have damaged tubes are more likely to have an ectopic pregnancy, but it isn't clear what causes it to happen.

MISCARRIAGE

A miscarriage is a devastating experience at any time. When it comes after years of infertility and treatment it is even harder to have to deal with, and reassurances that you can 'try again soon' may make you feel worse after it has taken so long to get this far.

The Human Fertilisation and Embryology Authority recognises that IVF pregnancies are slightly more likely to result in miscarriage than natural pregnancies. There are a number of factors which may explain this. Women who have had IVF treatment are more likely to be older than average, and miscarriages are more common in older women anyway. The fact that women who have had IVF treatment are more likely to be aware that they have had an early miscarriage may also play a part. It is quite possible that many women who have conceived naturally miscarry in the first few weeks before they have even realised that they were pregnant, and the miscarriage is seen as a late period.

Although up to a third of women will experience a miscarriage at some point in their lives, it isn't always clear what the cause is and as a rule tests are not done until a woman has miscarried three times. Early miscarriages are often caused by genetic problems with the foetus, which could never have developed properly either because of some deformity or because the placenta is not working. Sometimes the fertilised egg stops developing at an early stage while the placenta and sac continue to form. This is called an anembryonic pregnancy, or a blighted ovum, and is quite common. Most miscarriages happen before the twelfth week of pregnancy.

If you lose a baby after IVF treatment you will need help and counselling to help you cope with the bereavement process and to recognise your right to grieve for your loss. It may be helpful to contact the Miscarriage Association, who can give support and advice, and it is worth remembering that the vast majority of women who have had a miscarriage go on to have a normal pregnancy afterwards.

WHEN TREATMENT FAILS

It is a sad fact that most first IVF treatments will fail. The national figures show that on average about 15 per cent of treatment cycles are successful. If you get as far as embryo transfer your chances of getting pregnant will have improved, with an average live birth rate per embryo transfer of 19.5 per cent. Realistically, your chances of success are very much dependent on your age and circumstances. The live birth rate per treatment cycle for IVF in a woman between the ages of twenty-five and twenty-nine is above 18 per cent, but for a woman who is over forty-five it is just over 2 per cent. The IVF success rates drop sharply for women over forty unless they are using donor eggs.

Doctors cannot always explain why IVF hasn't worked. If the treatment cycle has gone well and the embryos have been good quality, there is often no clear reason why it doesn't result in a pregnancy. Some embryos don't implant and no one can explain why. Many women feel that their body, which has already failed to conceive naturally, has let them down again – but it is important not to blame yourself in these circumstances. The fact that there is no explanation merely serves to highlight the limitations of modern science, which is far from providing all the answers about the miracle of conception.

Just because your first treatment cycle has failed, this doesn't mean that IVF will not work for you. Many of those who have had successful IVF treatment have not succeeded initially. However, knowing this doesn't make it any easier if it happens to you.

When I found out my first IVF cycle hadn't worked I was surprised to feel a strange sense of relief. The tension and anxiety of the two-week wait was over at last. So it hadn't worked – but I hadn't in my heart of hearts expected it to. The whole thing had seemed impossible somehow: how could we expect a new person to grow from the tiny blobs we'd seen in the laboratory? Max had been certain it would work, and was extremely disappointed. For the first time, he started to wonder whether we might never have a child of our own.

I didn't want to talk about it at all for the first few days, and went around on a strange artificial high. I decided I would make the most of enjoying all the things I wouldn't have been able to do if we had children, so I went out every night and set about planning an exotic holiday. I was congratulating myself on how well I had coped with it all when a huge wave of gloom came crashing down and the reality of the treatment not working suddenly hit me. IVF had been our last and only chance. After all the years of waiting it was meant to be the solution to all our problems, the amazing high-tech treatment which would allow us to achieve what nature had denied. Now it had failed, there was nothing else left to try. This was as far as modern medicine went, and if we couldn't manage to make a baby with IVF then we'd never be able to. I couldn't talk about it without bursting into tears. I couldn't imagine it ever getting any easier, and I started to doubt whether I had the strength to start all over again.

It's only natural to feel depressed after an unsuccessful treatment cycle. You will have invested time and energy in your treatment, and just getting through it will have used up a lot of your emotional stamina. When IVF doesn't work you feel frightened that maybe nothing is ever going to work, and that maybe you will have to get used to the fact that you are not going to be able to have a child of your own – which is all the more painful after having had your hopes raised by going through the successive stages of the treatment cycle.

CHANGING CLINICS

It is very easy to blame the clinic if the treatment doesn't work. Some clinics are undoubtedly more successful than others, but a high success rate may have more to do with the patients being treated than with the medical expertise of the staff. An unsuccessful first IVF cycle can have an important diagnostic value, helping the medical team to understand more about your individual circumstances and enabling a second cycle to run more smoothly, with a greater chance of success. Familiarity with the staff, and their familiarity with your individual case, can be very important. These are all things worth considering before deciding to change to a new clinic, where the staff will need to start all over again. You may find a new team will want to repeat a lot of tests you have already been through and it can feel as if you are going right back to the beginning. Obviously, if you are unhappy with the treatment at your present clinic it would be foolish to stay there, but being swayed by one unsuccessful IVF cycle alone is not necessarily a good idea.

When our first treatment cycle didn't work, I immediately started wondering whether we might have had more chance of success at another clinic. I spent hours looking at all the statistics, and rang round hospitals collecting brochures and price lists. I became obsessed with success rates and even went to discuss the matter with my GP, who was very understanding but told me it could be counter-productive to change clinics, and that I couldn't expect to change every time a treatment cycle didn't work. We decided to give it another try at the same place, and when we did start again it was very helpful to be somewhere familiar with staff we knew and who knew us. It made the whole thing easier and much more relaxed.

HELP AND SUPPORT

After an unsuccessful treatment cycle, being part of a hospital support group or a self-help group can be invaluable. Only those who have been there themselves can genuinely understand how you are feeling, and just being with other people who know what it is like can be a great relief. The fertility organisations Child and Issue both have helplines for members and can provide support.

Telling friends and family that the treatment hasn't worked is another hurdle which has to be overcome. I found it very difficult to tell people at first because I couldn't bear to talk about it, and it's not the sort of thing you can drop easily into everyday conversation. I dreaded people being kind and feeling sorry for me because that made me feel sorry for myself, and I kept bursting into tears whenever anyone was nice about it.

It is hard for anyone to say the right thing at this stage, and you are going to feel irritated and annoyed by some people's reactions. So many of them seemed to want to give us cheering advice, reassuring us that it was bound to work next time and eagerly asking when we could start again. No one seemed to understand that it hadn't been easy, and had left us feeling drained and depressed. It was as if we had to forget it had ever happened and merrily dash off for another treatment cycle. There was no recognition of the emotional trauma involved in an unsuccessful attempt. We got upset by people who repeatedly asked what we were going to do next, as if we were bound to have some neat masterplan. For me the most annoying people were those who asked if we'd thought about fostering or adoption, reinforcing my doubts that I'd ever be able to become pregnant and have a child. People may say things which are incredibly hurtful when you are feeling so vulnerable, but try to remember that most of them have no idea how to deal with your situation and are at a loss as to what to say or do. They may be sad themselves that it hasn't worked for you, and are only trying to make you feel better, even if they aren't succeeding.

You will need time to recover emotionally after an unsuccessful treatment. I felt very upset about it for a while afterwards. Counselling may be useful at this time, even if you haven't seen a counsellor before. I decided I didn't want to see a counsellor, and was surprised that the clinic did not make my next appointment with the doctor until some weeks after the unsuccessful treatment. But in retrospect that was very sensible – had it been any earlier I would have been much too upset to talk logically about what to do next. As it was, I had started to feel much better by the time of the appointment, and we were able to have a sensible discussion about why the treatment might have failed and what we should do next.

Remember, it does get easier with time. It sounds incredibly trite when you are still feeling raw after unsuccessful treatment, but it does get better. Whatever you decide to do – whether to go ahead with more treatment, to change clinics, to forget about treatment and give yourself a breathing space for a while, or to consider other options – you will gain strength as time goes by.

TRYING AGAIN

Some people feel they want to try again as soon as they can, but you will have to wait a few months to allow your body to get back to normal.

The average success rates for IVF may seem very low at only 15 per cent, but this is the rate per treatment cycle. It may help to look at IVF as a course of treatment, rather than as a one-off last chance which will never work if the first attempt fails. Cumulative success rates for IVF can be surprisingly high: a 1992 study showed a live birth rate of around 70 per cent after four treatment cycles in couples where the woman is under forty and the man has normal sperm. Research at another hospital showed that 80 per cent of their patients had a baby over six attempts at IVF.

Most couples who have had a test-tube baby will have had more than one attempt at IVF before they succeeded. No one can say how many attempts you should have before you decide that IVF isn't going to work for you. Some couples may find one unsuccessful attempt so stressful that they decide not to put themselves through it again. Others will have numerous attempts before they either achieve success or decide to give up. Your doctors may advise you as to whether they think it is worth continuing after repeated unsuccessful attempts, but couples who can afford to try over and over again will always find clinics willing to treat them. Ultimately the decision is yours, and only you know how much you are prepared to go through.

HAVING A BREAK

Many couples find that taking a break from treatment at some stage can be refreshing. Time may help you to rethink your aims completely, and you may decide you don't want to go ahead with more treatment. Alternatively, you may feel ready to face your next IVF cycle with renewed vigour and optimism. Either way, taking some time out can be a positive step.

When you are going through repeated treatment cycles the rest of your life stands still and everything else takes second place. You are always either going through a treatment cycle, getting over it or waiting to start the next one. Some people say it feels as if they are in an endless tunnel, or a maze. All you want is an end and a solution, but however desperately you try nothing seems to get you any closer to that point.

When our first treatment cycle didn't work, I didn't know if I'd ever be able to face going through it all again. We were told we could try again in three months, but we ended up having a break of about six months, saving some money and going away. We had the sort of holiday we couldn't have contemplated if I'd been pregnant or we'd had a young child, and there was some small compensation in knowing that we were making the best of our situation. If this were the apocryphal old wives' tale we've all heard a thousand times, I would have discovered I was pregnant when I got home. Of course I didn't, and our next treatment cycle didn't work either, but getting away and having some time to ourselves did give us a breathing space and made us feel stronger about starting again.

HELPING YOURSELF

You can do a lot of things yourself to maximise your chances of success. Giving up smoking, eating healthily and not drinking too much alcohol can all have a positive effect and help you to feel better about yourself. Sometimes it may be worth thinking about other areas of your life which you could change, as reducing stress can only be a good thing. Some women find that their careers are their salvation during fertility treatment, but for others cutting back on their working hours or changing jobs may have a beneficial effect.

You put off so many other things when you are going through IVF – sometimes because all your money is being spent on treatment and you don't have any left for anything else, sometimes because you are waiting for an end to your ordeal before you get on with the rest of your life. Helping yourself to feel that you are moving forward in other ways is essential. Don't put off applying for promotion or a better job, cutting back your hours or giving up work. Trying to do what you want with the rest of your life, and making it as enjoyable as you possibly can at such a difficult time, will only make things better.

COMPLEMENTARY THERAPIES

With the current boom in complementary medicine many patients are choosing alternative therapies to treat a wide variety of problems and illnesses. Many of these therapies adopt a holistic approach, treating the mind and body as a whole, rather than isolating a part of the body which is not working properly and treating that alone.

Some people deny that complementary medicine can have any value at all in treating a long-standing fertility problem, and it is certainly true that a physical structural cause of infertility is not likely to be miraculously solved by alternative therapies. However, that doesn't mean there is no role for such treatments, particularly when they are used alongside modern medical methods.

Some couples find that complementary medicine can help them prepare for conventional treatment. It may improve their general health and wellbeing and make them feel more relaxed and positive. Many practitioners of complementary medicine feel that they can be most useful in sorting out subtle imbalances and restoring the body's natural harmony, and this may help as you go through conventional treatment. Some complementary therapists do claim successes in treating infertility, particularly where it is unexplained, but the evidence is largely anecdotal.

But before you investigate complementary medicine, a note of caution. It is vital to make sure that you are seeing a reputable therapist who is recommended by the appropriate professional body. You may want to check whether they have any experience in treating people with fertility problems. If you feel better after consulting a complementary therapist, if it is something which is helping you to feel healthier and generally better about yourself, then it is worth doing. But it can be easy to squander your savings on expensive private consultations with therapists who hold out a ray of hope, and some couples end up spending a small fortune trying every complementary treatment under the sun without success.

GIVING UP ON TREATMENT

For some patients IVF may provide a happy ending, but for others there will be different paths ahead. It can be very difficult to know when to give up, as there is the constant nagging doubt that you might not have tried every available avenue, and that one more treatment cycle at a different hospital, with a different doctor, or using a slightly different technique, might just work.

In some cases, where there is clear medical evidence that

further cycles are not likely to succeed, the clinic may advise a couple that it would be best to stop. It can be more difficult where a couple are producing good-quality embryos each time but they are failing to implant. Most clinics suggest trying three or four cycles, and thousands of couples go through a number of cycles before they succeed. Many have more than four cycles, but data from the Human Fertilisation and Embryology Authority suggests that the live birth rate falls significantly in those who make more than ten attempts. It can take a while to come to terms with the decision to give up on treatment, but it may bring with it an immense and sometimes unexpected sense of relief.

OTHER ROUTES TO PARENTHOOD

Fertility treatment isn't the only way to have a family: there are a number of other options you may wish to consider. None of them will offer easy or instant solutions and they will probably bring a whole new set of problems, but you may want to find out more about other ways of becoming parents.

Surrogacy

In surrogate parenthood another woman carries a pregnancy for a couple who cannot otherwise have a child of their own. In what is known as 'straight' surrogacy, the surrogate uses the male partner's sperm to inseminate herself. In 'host' surrogacy the couple produce their own embryo, using IVF techniques, which is then transferred into the surrogate. Straight surrogacy can be done by the surrogate and the couple themselves, but host surrogacy can obviously only be carried out through an IVF clinic.

Surrogacy is a controversial area, with potential hazards at every step. Trust between the couple who want the child, known as the 'commissioning couple', and the surrogate mother is essential. In the United Kingdom the commissioning couple have to adopt the child before it is legally theirs, and should the surrogate mother change her mind about giving up the child during the pregnancy or birth she has a legal right to do so. In the same way, if the commissioning couple decide that they don't want the child after all, the surrogate mother is legally responsible for it. Too much is left to trust in this arrangement, with commissioning couples terrified that the surrogate will decide she can't bear to part with the baby, and surrogate mothers worried that they may be left with a child they don't want. Some kind of binding legal contract has been suggested as one way to solve this problem.

The issue of payment for the surrogate is another problem. Currently, the commissioning couple may pay the surrogate reasonable expenses, but there is no definition of what this might mean. It can include travelling and medical expenses, ante-natal care and compensation to cover her time away from work.

Finding a suitable surrogate mother is probably the most difficult part of all. There is an agency in the United Kingdom which exists to help couples considering surrogacy. Founded by Kim Cotton, who was herself a surrogate mother, COTS, or Childlessness Overcome Through Surrogacy, provides information and practical help for couples who are considering surrogacy. A splinter group of COTS, called Triangle, matches couples with potential surrogates. Lists of couples looking for surrogate mothers are compiled and sent to women who are considering acting as surrogates, who can choose a couple they think they might like to help. The organisation says it has helped with more than two hundred surrogate births since it was founded, but claims the media focusses on the handful of cases which have gone wrong.

One of those was that of Karen Roche, who agreed to be a surrogate mother for a Dutch couple in return for payment. Karen Roche became pregnant, but soon she and the Dutch couple began to have doubts about each other and she told them she had terminated the pregnancy. The case hit the headlines, with both parties telling their side of the story and a lot of moral outrage. In a dramatic twist, it became apparent that Karen Roche had not had an abortion and was still pregnant. She said she had changed her mind about the surrogacy arrangement, and intended to keep the baby herself.

This sad story illustrated the way a surrogacy agreement can fall apart, causing deep distress and anguish to all concerned. The UK government announced a review of the law on surrogacy after the case aimed at tightening up the current arrangements.

Adoption

This is something which many couples consider when fertility treatment doesn't work. It is a permanent legal arrangement under which the child you have adopted becomes part of your family. The first and most important thing to understand before you think seriously about adoption as a possible way ahead is that in the UK it is very rare to find a baby who needs new parents (but see also Overseas Adoption, below). The vast majority of children who are adopted are older, and many have had difficult backgrounds or have special needs. They may not be easy children to look after, and you must be sure you really understand what you might be taking on before you consider this path. There are often strict age limits for prospective parents, and you may find that you fall outside these if you have already spent some time trying to have a child of your own and going through unsuccessful fertility treatment.

For couples who think they would like to try to adopt a child, the first step is to contact an adoption agency. There are about two hundred agencies in Britain and British Agencies for Adoption and Fostering can provide their details. Some are attached to local authorities while others are independent voluntary agencies. An agency will begin by sending you information about the way it works and the process you would go through should you decide to go ahead.

Adoption can be a long and difficult process, which may be even harder to cope with after years going through the fertility maze. Some professionals working in the field can be slightly wary of couples who come from this background, fearing that they might not be honest with themselves about whether they really want to adopt an older child, one who is emotionally disturbed or who has special needs. But as long as you are realistic about what you would be willing to deal with, this shouldn't be a problem.

Even so, the process will be drawn out as the agency will want to be absolutely certain that adoption is right for you before they approve you as prospective parents. There will be a lot of questions about your personal life and about what you are hoping for from adoption. A detailed assessment known as a homestudy is carried out by a social worker. There will be a series of interviews, and health, employment and police records will all be checked and evaluated before a written report is produced. It is important to understand that the adoption process focusses on the needs of the child and matching them to the right parents, not on the needs of the prospective parents.

Once a couple have been accepted as prospective parents, they can be matched with a child. This can take time and, even after a child has been placed with the prospective parents, it will be a while before the adoption is made legal in court.

Fostering

Done on a temporary basis, fostering involves looking after children who may eventually return to their own families. It is often necessary to help children through a difficult time when they cannot be with their parents, and fostering is an alternative to placing them in a children's home. The aim of successful fostering is to provide a happy short-term solution, not to create a family.

Sometimes people who foster children do so on a long-term basis when the child is not likely to return to his or her parents. These children may end up being adopted, or their family relationships may mean this is not an option.

Fostering is often short-term and uncertain, and could cause heartache for childless couples. The children who need foster carers may be difficult or disturbed. It can be hard to have all the responsibility of looking after them on a day-to-day basis, but no rights to make decisions. There may be great rewards in being able to help a child through a difficult time by offering a happy and supportive environment, but it can be emotionally demanding and it is not easy to be constantly aware that a child will eventually leave and return to his or her parents.

Overseas Adoption

For couples who are interested in adopting only a baby or a very young child, overseas adoption can seem an attractive alternative. Although it is not usually possible to adopt a newborn baby, some overseas countries allow abandoned children to be adopted before their first birthday. The age limits for parents vary from country to country, but older couples may find they are still allowed to adopt from overseas when they would not be considered as adoptive parents of UK children.

Overseas adoption has had a bad press in recent years with stories of babies being smuggled out of their birth countries and of unscrupulous agents selling children for illegal adoption. It is perfectly possible to adopt a child legally from overseas, but there is considerable controversy about this kind of trans-racial adoption. Some people claim that it can never be right to take children away from the country of their birth to bring them up in a different culture. They argue that resources should be put into enabling these children to live in better circumstances in their own countries rather than moving them overseas. If you are considering adopting from abroad you should be aware that you may encounter these arguments, and consider the implications carefully. Nowadays couples adopting from abroad are encouraged to embrace the culture of their child's birth country and to make sure they fully understand what they are embarking on by becoming a mixed family.

Many couples have managed to adopt from overseas success-fully, but it can be a lengthy and expensive business. One major problem for couples from the United Kingdom is that there is no agency dealing with overseas adoption, and prospective adopters have to make their own arrangements (though there is a support group: see below). The first step is to find a country which permits overseas adoptions. In some countries there is a state system for adoption, but in others there is no such framework and adoption lawyers have to be used. This is the stage when problems with illegal adoptions are most likely to occur, but they may be avoided by making sure you are using a lawyer who comes recommended by the country's consulate. In the same way as in the adoption of a British child, a home study is carried out to decide whether a couple would be suitable as adoptive parents, and this can be a prolonged and expensive business.

Once the couple have found a child abroad who needs a new family, they will have to go through the adoption process in his or her country of birth, which may involve a lengthy stay overseas. It may be necessary to adopt the child again in the UK, as the original adoption may not be recognised here.

If you are thinking about overseas adoption there is an organisation called OASIS which can help. It supports couples who are considering adopting from abroad, and can put you in touch with people who have adopted from particular countries.

CHILDLESSNESS

Some couples eventually decide to accept a future without children of their own. Living through years of infertility and treatments can make you negative about all aspects of your life. Things you used to enjoy often disappear in a quagmire of sadness as you focus on your desire for a child to the exclusion of everything else. Stepping off the treadmill may, with time, give you the opportunity to appreciate the good things you do have in your life.

Looking at a future without children is never going to be an easy thing to come to terms with, and may involve rethinking everything you have expected from life. Learning to cope with this is bound to be a painful process. Only those who have personal experience can really understand what it is like. Counselling may help, as can spending time with other couples who have decided not to pursue treatment or who have got further down the road of accceptance.

5

Success

A positive pregnancy test is what you have been dreaming of throughout what is likely to have been years of infertility, and it can be hard to believe at first. If you are fortunate enough to have a successful treatment cycle, finding out that it has worked will be one of the happiest moments of your life and one you will never forget.

I had decided to do a home pregnancy test on the day we were due to go to the clinic for our blood test after our last treatment cycle, because I couldn't bear the thought of getting the bad news that it hadn't worked from someone else over the telephone. I remember waking up very early and creeping off to the bathroom with my pregnancy testing kit, trying to brace myself for another disappointment. I sat and watched the kit as a blue line slowly appeared across one of the little windows, and then a second blue line in the other. I just presumed that meant it hadn't worked and carried on cleaning my teeth when it suddenly struck me that *two* blue lines meant it was positive. But instead of 'Hoorah, I'm pregnant!', my immediate thought was that there was something wrong with the test.

I went and had the blood test at the hospital as early as I could, and we spent the rest of the day waiting to find out whether that would be positive too. Max had already rung the clinic to ask them about our positive home test, and had been assured that it was most unlikely to be wrong. Even so, I was convinced there had been some kind of mistake until the hospital rang to tell me that the blood test too had shown I was pregnant.

It can be upsetting to discover that the pregnancy you have longed for brings with it a whole new set of problems and worries. The one thing you are experienced at by this stage is not being pregnant. Every time your period has started or you've had a negative pregnancy test it will have been sad and difficult, but it's something you've grown accustomed to dealing with. Finding yourself pregnant at last can be quite terrifying after the initial euphoria – you discover how scared you are that something might go wrong, that you might miscarry or that there might be some kind of medical problem. As there is a slightly higher rate of miscarriage in an IVF pregnancy, many women feel very nervous.

Many couples who conceive naturally wait until a pregnancy has passed the twelve-week stage, when the risk of miscarriage dwindles, to let other people know that they are expecting a baby, but you may find that you are denied this choice if you have told people about your treatment. Some couples are just so overjoyed that they tell everyone anyway, but if you do feel cautious about celebrating it can be difficult to have to tell other people so early in your pregnancy.

THE IVF PREGNANCY

You will probably have a scan or two at the fertility unit in very early pregnancy to check that everything is developing normally and to see how many of the embryos you had put back have implanted successfully.

We went back to the clinic for our first scan at six weeks. I was absolutely terrified that it would show I wasn't pregnant after all, as I still didn't have any of the symptoms of pregnancy I had spent so many years imaging. We were both quite overcome when the doctor turned the screen round to show us a little pulsating blob, which was our baby with its heart beating away.

We had a second scan at eight weeks, and already the changes in the embryo were apparent. It was much bigger and we could see the sac which would become the placenta. This was to be our last visit to the fertility clinic, and we felt a little sad as we left. Suddenly we were out in the world of pregnancy and birth all alone, and being treated like everyone else expecting a child. For most couples, finding out that they are expecting a baby is the beginning, but if you are expecting an IVF baby you feel that you have been through so much already that the difficult part ought to be over. I was lucky to have two very calm and calming midwives looking after me throughout my pregnancy. They managed to make me realise that, just because I had had a hard time getting pregnant, it didn't necessarily follow that I would inevitably have a hard time *being* pregnant.

However, many women do feel miserable during pregnancy. You may be very sick and tired and find it physically and emotionally difficult to cope with. Women who have conceived naturally tend to be more relaxed about admitting this and moaning about it, but if you are expecting a long-awaited baby you may feel under pressure to be constantly happy and bouncy. It will only make it worse if you don't appreciate that it is perfectly normal to feel less than marvellous at times during pregnancy, and to give in to that feeling.

Having been monitored so carefully throughout their fertility treatment, many women find it alarming not to get such close attention once they are pregnant. In early pregnancy you will often have a month between each ante-natal check, which can seem an eternity after your constant visits to the clinic during your treatment. I spent too much time reading books about pregnancy in between my ante-natal checks, and managed to convince myself that I had every possible complication. The best thing you can do at this stage is to try to relax and look after yourself. If you do have any specific worries you should not feel afraid to contact your midwife or doctor.

In your ante-natal classes, you may feel you have little in

common with the other pregnant women. I always used to feel everyone else was 'properly' pregnant, as if my bump was somehow not quite as real as theirs. Pregnancy is a new experience for everyone the first time around, but when your have waited so long for it to arrive it can seem even more extraordinary.

If you are open about how your baby was conceived, you may find that you are not the only one carrying an IVF baby. One of the women I used to sit next to in my ante-natal classes, and whose bump I had admired as one of those 'proper' ones, turned out to have conceived her baby by IVF too. We only discovered this once we had both given birth, but if either of us had mentioned it earlier we might have found it quite helpful!

THE MULTIPLE PREGNANCY

The medical team will be able to tell from the first scan at the fertility unit how many of the embryos you had transferred have implanted. If you had three embryos transferred and then have a positive pregnancy test, there is a 32 per cent chance of you having a multiple pregnancy. If you have had two embryos transferred the multiple pregnancy rate is 24 per cent.

A multiple pregnancy can seem like the answer to all your dreams, and many women have a perfectly happy and healthy pregnancy when they are carrying more than one baby, but there is a greater risk of complications. The main danger is of a premature delivery, which means the babies will weigh less and be more prone to difficulties with their breathing and blood supply and to have mental or physical disabilities. The miscarriage rate is higher in women who are carrying triplets, and sometimes one of the foetuses will be lost during pregnancy which can be very distressing.

If you are carrying more than one baby your pregnancy will be more closely monitored to check for raised blood pressure, anaemia, oedema and pre-eclampsia. You will be more likely to have your babies delivered by caesarean section than a woman carrying one child.

Coping with the demands of one small baby can be a shock to the system, but dealing with two or three can be very hard to manage and you will need all the help and support you can get. Twins or triplets will also mean you have to buy two or three of everything, and it can be a very expensive business. The Twins and Multiple Births Association offers encouragement and support to parents both before and after multiple births, and its help can be invaluable. As so many multiple births nowadays are the result of fertility treatment, TAMBA has a special infertility support group to help parents who've had treatment and can put you in touch with others who have had similar experiences.

THE IVF BIRTH AND AFTER

Some consultants are much more cautious about the birth of an IVF baby than they are when dealing with a baby which has been conceived naturally. When I was pregnant I read three separate magazine articles about women expecting IVF babies who were induced on their due dates 'for safety's sake', rather than being allowed to go into labour naturally. Unless you have had other problems, or are carrying more than one baby, you shouldn't still be thinking of yourself as different when it comes to the birth itself. The only thing which may make your baby's birth different is the fact that you have been waiting a lot longer than most other women, so it will be extra-special when it finally happens.

The experience of infertility never entirely leaves you, even after the birth of your baby. The pain and hurt disappear, and going through treatment again for a second child will never be as difficult, but you will inevitably be a different person because of what you have been through. Once you do emerge on the other side you will probably find that you are both stronger and wiser, and you will always feel an incredible empathy with those who are still struggling to find a way out of the fertility maze.

6

Experiences of IVF

The stories which follow are based on a series of in-depth interviews with the nine couples concerned. They talked honestly and openly about events which had often been traumatic and upsetting at the time, and were willing to rake over painful feelings from the past in the hope that other couples still stuck in the fertility maze might be able to gain strength from reading their stories. Some have asked for their names to be changed to protect their identities, as not all of their friends, families and colleagues are aware of their situations.

Their experiences cover a wide range of problems, situations and outcomes. They deal with male and female infertility, egg donation, sperm donation and intra-cytoplasmic sperm injection (ICSI). Some of the couples have been successful and now have children. Others are still having treatment, or have decided not to continue with IVF. Some of their experiences are harrowing, all are inspiring.

These couples are not in any way intended to be representative, as everyone's experience of infertility, of tests and of treatment will be unique. The stories they tell may be very different from yours, particularly as they cover some of the extreme circumstances which can arise. However, they do offer a very wide-ranging picture of IVF today, and I hope that

everyone will be able to find some common ground and to gain
something from their experiences.

SARAH AND PAUL'S STORY

'I felt I was sitting on the sidelines of my life watching it go
by, with absolutely no control over anything. I couldn't
play any part in it at all.'

**Sarah and Paul live near Great Yarmouth in Norfolk. They
met at the oilfield services company where they both work.
Sarah is thirty-one and Paul thirty-four. They had three
unsuccessful donor insemination attempts because of
Paul's low sperm count, before they were told that ICSI
might be the solution to their problems. Sarah is now
pregnant after their third attempt at ICSI.**

Sarah: Paul and I are both divorced. We were both drifting
along in useless marriages when we found each other and
became happy again. That was a good start. I felt in my previous
marriage that I wasn't ready for children. I couldn't say why –
whether it was because I wasn't happy enough or because I
didn't see my partner as a father and I didn't trust him.

When Paul and I got together it was pretty instant, really. I
came off the Pill about six months down the road. I thought
there was hardly any danger of me falling pregnant. I knew that
in Paul's previous marriage he had problems. His wife was
hounding him to get treatment, and he went along with it
because it was what she wanted.

Paul: We'd been doing tests for a couple of years. They couldn't
say why my sperm count was low. They thought that perhaps I'd
had mumps when I was a baby, or something like that. I thought
the sperm were so bad that there was nothing they could do
about it.

Sarah: I decided what I wanted and I spoke to Paul about it, and
he seemed a bit non-committal at first. If you've got a problem

on your side like that it must be difficult, but I said there was no way I was prepared to go through what we thought was to be IVF on my own – mentally, not just physically. I said if he didn't want to do it I could live with that, but I wasn't prepared to do it on my own. With that, he crawled out of his shell and said, 'No, no, let's talk about it.'

Paul and Sarah decided to go ahead with tests at their local hospital, hoping that they would be offered IVF.

Sarah: It's most peculiar the way they treat you. Paul had to go to the hospital, and then I had to go separately, and then finally they'd get the results together. They don't treat you as a couple. A lot of the tests have to be done at certain times of the month, particularly on the woman. Everything seemed to take an eternity.

Paul: That was the worst bit of all – the waiting at the local hospital.

Sarah: We saw the consultant, who said that Paul's sperm count was awful. He didn't know why. He said that IVF wasn't for us, and our only way forward was donor insemination. He never suggested anything about ICSI, or even told us that it existed.

The consultant suggested a private hospital. We'd actually had some of the investigative tests done there, because they were covered by our health insurance at work. We don't know if it had brought things forward or not, but whenever possible we'd had tests done privately.

We left it several months and then I asked them for their price list. Donor insemination was considerably cheaper than IVF. Since we'd been told IVF wasn't any good for us anyway, all we could do was think we'd saved ourselves a lot of money.

Sarah and Paul decided to start treatment at the hospital, using donor sperm.

Sarah: Paul's outlook is that if choice is taken away from you, you knuckle under. You can't sit there and say, 'I'm too proud to have a donor insemination baby', because you don't have a choice – or you don't think you have a choice.

The selection of the donor was done on eye colour, hair colour, blood group, build and general physical characteristics. On one occasion, on the day of the insemination they said they could only match some of the characteristics. You could request the same donor each time, but they are only allowed to donate a limited number of times. Also, if you had a child and later they wanted to get married, you could ring up and someone would check on the register to find out if they were related to the person they wanted to marry. But that's the only thing you could ask, and that's the only information you could ever find out.

They do the insemination in a completely natural cycle. You had to use an ovulation kit. I wanted someone to help me with that, really, but it seemed that everything was down to you to get the timing right.

They make the sperm do a swim test and only the strongest get selected. They just put the sample in a plastic catheter, feed it up inside you, squeeze, and that's it, they've gone. It's a bit like embryo transfer. They make you lie there for ten minutes and then you're allowed home.

They try for two or three cycles, and if it doesn't work I was told they give you Clomid or something like that to stimulate the ovaries.

Paul: They did the insemination twice, once right near the time of ovulation and then the following day or the day after to make sure they got it right.

I didn't feel involved – I just tagged along. In fact it was difficult for both of us to leave work at the same time. I did go with Sarah on one of the occasions we tried, but there wasn't much point in me being there. All I could do was stand and watch.

Sarah: We were split on whether we'd tell a child as they grew up. I said yes because I've always been a really forthright sort of person, but Paul said no. I think it's a very difficult decision. At what age would you tell a child? How would they take it? How would they understand? I think I would have just told them. There's no way they'd ever find their real father – they can't find out anything about them. But how would it make Paul feel if he wasn't the real father, even though he'd be the legal father?

Sarah and Paul had three unsuccessful attempts at donor insemination before they ran out of money and decided to stop.

Paul: We'd moved and we hadn't been in the house very long. We had to spend seven or eight thousand quid on windows and various other things. We had no choice – we had to spend money on the house, and then save a bit and spend it on fertility treatment. You can't have it all ways.

Sarah: To be stressed out and have someone taking your money away at the same time was just a bit too much. You know what it's like in a new house – you want to spend some money and make it your little home. For the last five years our jobs have been a bit shaky, so we've always made sure that we've saved up for something before we've bought it. But it does leave you feeling awfully tight, and as if you can't do anything. You can't even go out to dinner to cheer yourself up, because you're broke. That's what brought the donor insemination to an end.

Sarah had been given the number of a fertility counsellor, who told her that it might be possible for them to have further treatment paid for by the local health authority.

Sarah: I was told that the NHS might provide one free IVF cycle. When I spoke to the counsellor, it was coming in the next few months. That gave us new hope, even though we'd been told IVF wasn't for us.

Every Monday I'd ring the health authority hassling them about this money and asking whether it had been released yet. Finally they said yes, but you had to be put forward by your GP. Our GP was very good and put our names forward straightaway.

Sarah and Paul's local health authority had a contract with a teaching hospital in London which provided IVF treat-

ment. They were amazed to be told at their first appointment that they could be treated using a technique called ICSI, which is designed to help in cases where the man has a low sperm count. Under the system operating in Norfolk they could have the routine part of the cycle done locally, travelling to London for egg collection and embryo transfer.

Sarah: Because the London hospital sees so many patients from Norfolk they have rooms above a doctor's surgery in Norwich. There's a consulting room and office, a waiting room and a scan room.

There was very much the feeling that, instead of being worked on as two single people with separate reproductive cycles, we were worked on as a couple. We were invited as a couple. Our appointment was for both of us to go together.

The London end was all very well handled. When we first went to see the consultant they gave us loads of information about what would happen. They seemed much more clued up than our local hospital, where they were just running bits of tests and seemed all over the place.

I'm not a bitter person, but I do feel going to the consultant at the local hospital cost us about eighteen months. If he'd told us about ICSI we certainly would have started saving towards it, and we wouldn't have had the donor insemination. We never saw the consultant all the way through the tests – we just suddenly saw him for this grand appointment at the end. When we came out I asked Paul if he thought we should get a second opinion, but we didn't because we thought he was a qualified man who knew what he was talking about.

Paul and Sarah started their first ICSI cycle, paid for by the health authority.

Sarah: The treatment wasn't too bad. Paul did the injections at home for me so we didn't have to go to the surgery.
Paul: I was a bit apprehensive about doing the injections, but

once I'd done the first one it was OK. It didn't make me feel sick or anything until one day I pulled the needle out and a load of blood followed. I thought, 'What do I do now?'

Sarah: I was surprised that Paul just did the injections. He didn't seem to have any qualms about it at all. If you catch a capillary or whatever, you have to take the needle out and do it again. You get this trickle of blood straight down your leg and it's quite frightening. Fortunately it doesn't happen very often.

I've got the beginnings of polycystic ovarian disease. That's my only problem, and it didn't show up until they started giving me all the stimulation drugs. I had millions of eggs and they had to be careful not to overstimulate.

They said the egg collection was done under local anaesthetic, but as far as I was concerned it was general. They put a needle in my hand, and then I don't remember anything at all. I woke up not knowing the first thing that had happened, so I asked Paul because he had been sitting there with me.

Paul: You can't really see the screen that the guy is looking at because it's at an angle. I just looked at Sarah, held her hand, stroked her head and talked to her. And when she kicked her leg up I put it back down again.

Sarah: It was nice that Paul was there. It stops the man being so cut off from the process, and when I came round he could tell me what had happened.

I had a really rough egg collection the first time. I don't know what the doctor had done, but he left the hospital shortly afterwards. I was staying at my father's, about ten miles outside London. When I got back I just went to bed, and if I moved at all I couldn't breathe. The only reason I didn't call the hospital was because I was all right if I lay still.

I just wasn't aware that that wasn't how it should be. So I didn't make a fuss about it, and the second time I was expecting the same thing again. But that time the consultant did it, and afterwards, instead of being in bed I was in the garden dead-heading roses! I felt a bit sore, but fine in myself.

We had about nineteen eggs the first time, and seventeen were usable. We had donor back-up that time. They decided to put twelve eggs with Paul's sperm and five with the donor sperm. They said that gave the greatest chance to Paul's sperm. Out of the twelve, only one fertilised. We ended up with one of Paul's and three of the donor's.

We had a hell of a dilemma – whether to put back the one of Paul's or the three of the others. I said I hadn't gone through all that to have somebody else's sperm fertilise the eggs. Paul's was the best of the lot, and I reckoned I could go and do donor insemination any time.

We were talked into having donor back-up because Paul's sperm count was so low. They couldn't bear the idea of putting all the eggs with Paul's sperm and having none of them fertilise, and then having to tell us there were no embryos to put back into my womb.

Our embryo transfer was always done at a different private clinic. The hospital we went to doesn't do ICSI. They told us that after somebody has trained for IVF it takes a further two years to become ICSI-trained. The hospital buys in a service for ICSI from a private fertility clinic.

Once my eggs had been taken out at the hospital, Paul would have to take them over to the private clinic.

Paul: They give you the eggs in a sort of mini-oven set at the right temperature, and then they call a taxi for you – that's all part of the package. All the taxi drivers knew what was going on – they'd obviously done the trip many times for many different people. They'd say, 'Oh, you've got some eggs,' and I was thinking, 'I hope we don't crash.'

You go to the private clinic and you hand over the eggs to the embryologist. Then you go and do a sample and give it to the nurse. You go back to the hospital, while the people at the clinic put the eggs with the sperm to fertilise them.

Sarah: The clinic smacks of private treatment – you walk in and the carpet is about three inches deep. But the hospital was an awful lot better.

The first time we went to the private clinic to have the embryos put back it was unbearably hot in the waiting room, and we were in there for two hours. In all that time no one came and told us what was happening. I think that was awful.

The treatment at the hospital seemed a lot more personal. You tended to see the same people when you got there. They realised you had to travel some distance and wherever possible they gave you appointments later in the day, which helped with fares and that sort of thing.

The travel was just something else tacked on. We seriously wondered about their sanity at first when we found out that the treatment took place in London.

Paul: There's a day in between egg collection and embryo transfer, and we decided Sarah was going to stay at her Dad's in Essex. I'd be up at five in the morning, at the time of day when you're feeling your worst, and drive her there. I had to come back because of the dog. I'd go to work the next day and then drive back and pick her up again.

Sarah: If you had to go to London for the scans as well it would be unbearable. It's nicer to go on the train because you can just sit and relax, but we couldn't afford it. The standard train fare from Yarmouth to London is £57. There are cheaper tickets if you go later in the day, but all the ICSI appointments are first thing in the morning. If we wanted to go by train for the two days, it would be £228.

Sarah and Paul's first cycle of treatment was unsuccessful.

Sarah: We didn't expect I'd fall pregnant on the first treatment. It was a bit of a disappointment, but we'd had so much disappointment over the previous three years that it wasn't a surprise. Originally we said we'd go for three attempts. I said if I was going to do it at all I had to try it at least three times, and I wouldn't set about it just for one attempt.

Paul tends to be the pessimist and I tend to be the optimist, but they give you these statistical chances and when you get to the true figures, the live births per cycle, some of them are frighteningly low. They massage the statistics – there are so many different ways of writing them down.

Statistically we were quite young, and there was nothing wrong on my side. If we got to embryo transfer, which we did every time, they said there was a one-in-four chance. That seemed huge.

The couple saved to pay for a second treatment cycle privately at the same hospital, which they had as soon as they could, just three months later.

Sarah: The second time we again went along with what they suggested, and had donor back-up. Paul's sperm fertilised more eggs. We ended up with seven embryos that were viable, and they put three back.

The pregnancy test was due to be done on a Wednesday morning. On Tuesday nights Paul always goes to play darts. I said I didn't want to go because I didn't feel very well. I lay on the sofa watching television and all of a sudden I got a period pain. I went upstairs to check, and I was bleeding.

Paul: This second time I took the attitude that if I thought it wasn't going to work perhaps I wouldn't be so disappointed. But it doesn't work that way. You still feel disappointed.

Sarah: I'm a really practical person and so is Paul, but this really pushed us to our limits. The first cycle wasn't so bad, and with the second we thought it would be better because we knew how it went. But suddenly it was as if our whole lives had ground to a standstill. I'd had enough. I almost wanted to stop doing it entirely and forget about it for a little while.

I think the worst thing has been the length of time it's been going on. We've become increasingly short of money, which means you can neither do things to the house nor go out and enjoy yourself. Everything was centred around conserving money and the next trip to London.

I was also screwing up at work. The worst of it is the mental stress, which is a combination of the physical treatment with the drugs, the waiting and not having any money.

I don't think I'd have got through it without being able to talk to people – but some people, especially people with young children, just didn't know what to say. Apart from people that were close to me, I didn't want anything to do with other people's babies, bumps and pushchairs. You'd walk past the children's clothes in places like Woolworth's, places you'd go anyway, as if you had a blindfold on one side of your head. If you saw a pretty little dress or something like that, you had to put it right out of your mind.

Someone said to me 'You've got to get it out of your mind, put it out of your mind,' but that really is easier said than done. Have you ever sat and watched the telly and tried not to see a baby? There's babies everywhere. I came home that evening and I saw a Fairy ad, which has a baby on it, a Comfort ad which had some baby being wrapped up in a towel, and then something else. I hit the 'off' button because it was really getting on my nerves. Everybody loves to speak about babies, don't they? They're in your face all the time and you can't put it out of your mind just like that. Society doesn't let you. Society loves babies.

Paul: You'd go out shopping and you'd see some scruffy bloke, about six foot tall, and he'd have three kids and you'd think 'Why him and not me?' There's nothing you can do.

I'd talk to the blokes at work about it. They'd listen and they'd understand that it's just one of those things.

Sarah and Paul started their third ICSI cycle as soon as they could, again paying for the treatment.

Sarah: We'd done the three cycles consecutively, and by the third one I was like another person. I was in dreamland. I felt I was sitting on the sidelines of my life watching it go by, with absolutely no control over anything. I couldn't play any part in it at all. One day would just drift into another. I'm a normal person, but it was turning me into something else.

The third time I said I didn't want donor back-up. I said I could go and have donor insemination done whenever I chose for a lot less money. I just thought we'd be giving Paul's sperm a better chance if we put all the eggs with his sperm. They asked if we were sure. I made a big thing of saying I was sure and crossing out the donor back-up line on the form.

We had nineteen eggs, and twelve fertilised. The hospital

suggested freezing five, which was paid for by the NHS – which I found quite odd because we weren't on an NHS cycle.

We actually got to go and see the embryos – it makes everything a bit more of a reality. Otherwise, all you go through is a series of medical procedures and, although you know there's life involved there somewhere, you never see it. We had to take our shoes off before they let us into the lab. The lab people put them so we could see the three embryos together – they were about eight cells. It was weird to think that a baby grows from such a tiny thing.

Two weeks later it was time for the pregnancy test.

Sarah: I did the test on a Wednesday, a fortnight after the embryo transfer. There was a very faint line, but you had to look hard to see it and it certainly wasn't blue. This was at the crack of dawn, about six o'clock. The clinic was open at that time, so I phoned them up because I didn't know what else to do. I said, 'There's this line, but it's really faint and I don't think it's positive.' The nurse said if there was any sort of line I should stay on the drugs and do another test on the Friday.

We had all that time, from Wednesday to Friday, to wait. On Thursday nights I go to college, and as I was driving home I saw a shooting star up in the sky. I tend to be superstitious, but that just made me laugh because I thought it was ridiculous and no one would believe me if I told them.

When I woke up in the morning I did the test, and there it was, blue as day. I thought, 'What's the matter with it? What can have affected it?' I wasn't excited or anything. I called the clinic again and I asked, 'These tests – what can make them go wrong?'

The nurse replied, 'What do you mean, wrong? Is it positive?'

I said, 'Well, it looks positive.'

She said, 'Well, that usually means that you're pregnant.'

I said, 'No. The hormones and everything – what can make it go wrong?'

And she said, 'Nothing, really.'

She said I could go in and have another test done there, and in fact I'd arranged to take that day off because I was so fed up. I didn't really believe it. As I put the phone down, I thought, 'Oh, I might be pregnant.' It had suddenly dawned on me. I sat there and didn't dare move.

Paul was still asleep in bed. I made him a cup of coffee, then went back upstairs and put the test against his cup. He picked it up and looked at it and then said, 'It looks positive. What's the matter with it?'

Paul: You're so used to thinking that they're all going to be negative that when you get one that's right you just think, 'What's wrong with that, then?'

The test at the clinic confirmed that Sarah was pregnant and carrying one baby.

Paul: I'm looking forward to it. I'll just be glad when it turns up, when we've actually got the baby. I think you tend not to believe it until you've actually got the baby in your arms.

Sarah: I don't think it's really sunk in yet. I can't imagine myself having a baby. You can't believe it, can you? It's a peculiar feeling.

I've seriously thought about going through an egg donation cycle later on because I have so many eggs. I'll see how we go after the baby. When we found out I was pregnant I felt so sorry for all those people who were still trying.

I know I lost sight of the hope that I'd ever fall pregnant. You're given all these statistics and you don't listen to them because you become so down about it all. If they're telling you there's a chance, then there is, but you tend to overlook that. I wanted to run into the waiting room and say, 'Look, it can work. My man's got an awful sperm count and it worked. Try not to give up hope.'

When we got to the end of the third cycle I was ready to chuck in the towel. My whole self had been changed by it all. You forget that what you're going through is for a reason. You lose sight of the objective and wonder what the hell you're doing. It runs your life, it messes everything up. But try not to give up

hope because there is a chance. I'd do it again. If I felt I wanted
another child, I'd do it again.

DEBBIE AND TOM'S STORY

'Infertility treatment is an industry – an industry that's
founded on hope. All the talk is about "We can make this
happen." . . . You are sold this fantasy that you're going to
do it, and it's going to work.'

**Debbie is a civil servant and Tom works in information
technology. They are both in their thirties. They have had
four unsuccessful attempts at IVF, and have decided they
will try to adopt a child from overseas.**

Debbie: After about six months of trying we started talking to
people and they told us not to worry because it often takes a while.
I was thirty-one at the time, so I thought maybe it was my age.
After about eight or nine months we went to the doctor, and he
said, 'Don't worry. Come back in a year.' We went back a year later
and he referred us to our local hospital. We did all the tests there.
Tom: When we were doing the tests we had to do that post-
coital test – the worst of them all. They saw Debbie afterwards,
and the nurse told her that there were absolutely zero sperm.
Debbie: The first thing the nurse said to me was, 'Does your
husband smoke?', and I said no. She was looking terribly worried, and I asked what was wrong. She said she was sorry, but she
couldn't find a single sperm.

We've since discovered that when they do that test they often
find no sperm. But she didn't say to me, 'I don't know what this
means', or 'I've seen this happen before', or 'It probably means
nothing. Would you like an early appointment with the consultant?' It was awful. Out we went without anyone to talk to, no
doctors, nothing.
Tom: We didn't have an appointment with the consultant for
about four weeks. It was devastating. I felt that I was totally

infertile. I went and sat in the car and sobbed for about half an hour. I was destroyed by the whole thing. It wasn't until we went back weeks later that they confirmed it was rubbish.

Debbie: They did a load of tests and said that I was fine, but that Tom's sperm was not of fantastic quality. However, they said it was perfectly good enough to do various treatments, so we should go and see the people in their fertility unit. Off we went, and they said we should do intra-uterine insemination, which we did twice unsuccessfully.

Meanwhile, I was on the waiting list for a laparoscopy to double-check their results. They said they didn't need to do a laparoscopy, but they put me on the waiting list. The laparoscopy took place eleven or twelve months after the initial investigation. It turned out that I was severely scarred inside, and my fallopian tubes were completely blocked. It was a huge shock, having thought that I was all right.

I'd built up an assumption in my head about the way I was. I was completely zonked from the anaesthetic and they woke me up and this doctor came in – nobody I'd ever seen before – and just told me.

Tom: It was very brutal, but I don't know if there's any other way for them to do it. They didn't have our history. He just said that the tubes were blocked, it was bad news, and there was nothing they could do.

Debbie: I found it slightly easier when I knew there was something wrong with both of us. I had a tendency when it was just Tom to think, 'I'm fine.' Not that I wanted to go off with anybody else who could give me good sperm, but I was a bit angry with Tom about it – like it was his fault. When I found out that what was wrong with me was far more serious than what was wrong with Tom it was a really humbling experience for me, and I think it was a relief for Tom.

Tom: Prior to that I just felt totally guilty. It was easier when I knew that Debbie had problems as well. A lot of people asked if I felt it was my fault, but I never did. I felt that we were so committed to it together that, even though I knew I had the problem, I didn't feel it was going to break us apart.

Some people enquired whether I felt less of a man, but it makes no difference at all – that wasn't an issue. All sorts of odd assumptions were made. One friend remarked, 'So you're shooting blanks, are you?' I've never forgiven him. No one has ever said anything as tactless as that.

Debbie and Tom were told that they should try IVF, but their doctor refused to pay for any more drugs.

Tom: We got the drugs for the IUI, but they were redundant cycles because of Debbie's blocked tubes. By the time we came round to IVF they just said that was it, and they weren't funding us any more. I wrote to the hospital and said that they were responsible for wasting the money, but no one was interested. *Debbie*: They said it was our choice to continue with the IUI treatment. We wrote back and said that we'd done so on the advice of the consultant that it was the applicable treatment, but they refused to accept any responsibility.

When you're thirty-two, a year of your fertile life is a long time, and we'd wasted a year, lots of money and a lot of emotional stress.

Tom: We wanted to find out if we qualified for any funding for the IVF, and we did. We were fortunate enough to meet our local health authority's criteria and we did have one cycle funded. *Debbie*: But we still had to pay for all the drugs, which cost a fortune – about £800 a cycle.

Tom: I just took it on the chin that they were going to be like this, but then I found out that other GPs not far away would fund the drugs. Doctors don't necessarily see infertility as an illness. They don't see it as critical that you have this treatment. *Debbie*: That's something I found difficult about the whole thing. Infertility is seen as an optional illness. It's defined in the medical dictionary and by the World Health Organisation as a disease, like cancer or leukaemia, but it's an optional illness when it comes to money. I find that outrageous. I don't have cancer, I don't have anything else wrong with me – my personal illness is infertility.

There's funding for thousands of abortions. Not that I think people shouldn't have abortions, but our consultant at the hospital said that they'd pay to destroy a life but not to create one.

Tom: You can go and have loads of abortions. There's no limit on that.

Debbie and Tom went ahead with their first IVF cycle at the clinic, paying for the drugs themselves.

Debbie: I had slight ovarian hyperstimulation. I was very distended, and very uncomfortable. I had something like seventeen eggs collected, which was a huge number. They fertilised fifteen of them, but they said they wouldn't continue treatment because they were worried about me, so they froze them all.

Then we did the next cycle, and they defrosted them and only four survived, which we both felt a bit angry about. It didn't work.

Then we did yet another cycle from scratch. When we did the first cycle, the nurse did the injections in the clinic at eight in the morning, but the second time they taught us how to do it ourselves, and Tom did it. I could do it myself, but I didn't like doing so.

Again, there were quite a lot of eggs. I've got polycystic ovaries so it's very difficult to get the drug dosage right. I either had lots of eggs or not very many, but we always had excellent embryos.

Debbie and Tom's second attempt was also unsuccessful.

Debbie: I carried on going to work, and on the day I did the pregnancy test and it was negative I felt desperate. I went into the office. I'm a civil servant and I was writing a very serious letter. I realised when I was sitting on the train on the way home that I'd written absolute gobbledygook. I didn't even know what I was doing.

I got home and just collapsed. I couldn't stop crying, and I didn't go to work for about three weeks. I went to see the doctor, who said that she'd been waiting for me to come in. She had two other women doing IVF: both of them had already stopped going to work and had collapsed with the stress, and one of them was on anti-depressants. She said she'd been wondering how on earth I was managing to go on for so long. She said she'd give me as much time off work as I needed, and that the next time I did a treatment she'd sign me off and I could say whatever I wanted about why I wasn't there. That was great.

Debbie and Tom decided to try again at the hospital.

Tom: We were about to start the third cycle when they said that they were going to close the unit down. But they got an extension and managed to get everybody through. Working seven days a week, they rushed about thirty people through in a matter of weeks. It was ghastly – terribly rushed.

Debbie: On that cycle we had even more drugs. They said they'd rather I took the ones I'd previously taken as suppositories in the form of an injection, because it was more certain. It was an intra-muscular injection with a large needle. So I was having injections in my thighs every day, and then Tom was giving me this intra-muscular injection in my bum.

I actually lost sensation in my right thigh, and a year later I still haven't fully recovered it. I went to my GP who said it was the IVF injections – I'd hit the surface nerves, but my feeling would come back. She said it just happened sometimes, especially if you are inexperienced.

I've taken needles into meetings and gone to the loo, and I've taken them on trains and into hotels. I've sniffed in the middle of an important meeting at work. I had to go into a corner and sniff and say it was for a cold. It's quite funny because I'm sure there are a lot of people who know what you are doing. You know that they know.

Tom: It's extraordinary when you get on the network. Before we did we had no idea of the scale of the problem. Then you suddenly realise, once you start talking about it, quite how many people like you there are out there.

Debbie and Tom's third attempt didn't work, and by this time the unit where they'd been having treatment had closed down.

Debbie: After number three, I told Tom I didn't know if I could do it again. We took about six months off. We talked about it and rowed about it. If I'd had a choice I probably would have stopped at three, but I decided to give it one more try. I really did it for Tom, but I knew it would be the last time.

Tom: A lot of people whom we'd spoken to said if it's not working at one clinic, try somewhere else. It was fortuitous for us that our own clinic closed down. We went to a private hospital and they raised some other issues.

Debbie: There were three things that they thought it might have been, and they checked them. All of them showed that my womb was in very good shape, and my hormone levels were normal.

They did a scan and they thought I had a fibroid, which they were going to take out. When they put me under anaesthetic they discovered I did have a fibroid but it wasn't affecting my womb and it was fine, which I was very relieved about.

Tom: Going to a new hospital raised our hopes. They were much more organised, but actually it was very similar. They did the same thing, though with a slightly different mixture of drugs. But people say just a nuance can make a difference.

Essentially, it's all about whether or not you get a good embryo. If you get good eggs and sperm that's it, and the rest is down to nature. I felt both hospitals had done all that they could do because they'd got superb embryos, and beyond that there's nothing they can do.

Debbie: For me, taking the drugs, having the scans, the egg collection and all of that was much easier at the private hospital. I felt much better throughout the process.

The anaesthetist there is the best I have ever had. I react very badly to anaesthetic – it hits me very heavily, and I take a long time to recover. They do the egg collection there under general anaesthetic. Tom went out when I had it done, because he thought I'd be out for three or four hours after the operation. But I was already awake in the recovery suite, and by the time they took me back up to the bed I was up and reading. I felt fantastic.

At the first hospital they did the egg collection under heavy sedation – but that was heavier than the general anaesthetic! There I'd often come out of sedation midway through collection. They'd put me back under, but I'd felt intense pain as they'd collected the eggs.

Tom: I was much more involved at the original hospital, which had been really nice. I could go down to the operating theatre with Debbie, although I couldn't go in because of health and safety regulations. The nurse would bring the eggs out to the embryologist who was just the other side of the corridor. That was brilliant because I could see how the whole thing was going, I got to know the embryologist and I was much more involved in the whole thing.

At the private hospital I had no idea which part of the building Debbie was in for the egg collection. She was just whisked away, and then brought back.

Debbie: The one thing I really didn't like about the private hospital took place when we had the embryos replaced there. It was as if they were all off to a party, though I think they were trying to make us relax. They were saying, 'Hi, how are you? Lie down. Bring those embryos in.'

We'd been told at the original hospital that embryos have to be kept in a slightly darkened room, because they don't like the light. I asked the doctor, 'Why have you got all the lights on?' and he asked what I meant. When I told him he said, 'Oh, they don't know what they're doing at that hospital.'

Then they were talking about the Bahamas, and as they were putting the embryos in he asked if we'd ever been there. This moment is our equivalent of conception. This is the moment when you may or may not be making life, and he was standing there saying, 'Can you imagine yourself on the beach now?'

Tom: I hated him. It cheapened the whole thing. He was detestable.

Debbie and Tom's IVF cycle at the private hospital didn't work. They had already decided this would be their last try.

Debbie: We said at the beginning we'd do it four times, because there's a one-in-four chance, but we had no idea at that stage what we were doing or how it was going to be. The first time you don't know what you're doing, you're so busy working through the process that you're not really having the feelings that go with it. The next time you're slightly more familiar with the process so you can have more of the feelings, and it's actually more difficult. Then the next time you can do it with your eyes closed and you feel awful. The fourth time, because we were at an excellent private hospital which made the process so simple, I was aware only of how awful it was.

Tom: Debbie was keener to stop it than I was. I felt I had another one or two cycles in me. It was easier for Debbie to set a limit than for me, because it's not as punishing for the man as it is for the woman. I found it harder to let go of the process.

After the last cycle I came down with the most awful illness – a raging temperature which was purely stress-related. I lost half a stone in three days, and I couldn't leave the house for nine days.

Because Debbie had to go through all the physical processes of each cycle I would support her emotionally and do everything else for her – be at the hospital as much as I could, do the washing and the cleaning, the whole lot. Emotionally, I was more concerned with looking after Debbie than with looking after myself. At the end I had so neglected myself that I just collapsed. I was very, very depressed.

I had peaked with depression and exhaustion, but I felt a tremendous sense of relief that it was over. We'd already been thinking for a long time about other options, including overseas adoption. There's something so attractive about moving on to an area where we can have some control. With time and money and energy, we can probably make adoption happen. That's quite a positive position to be in. It's exactly four years since we started trying for kids, four years of disappointment and four years of negative experiences. We started doing lots of research about overseas adoption, and it's not as rosy as all that, but there's some glimmer of hope that we can have a family.

Debbie: There's a massive grieving process about the loss of your dreams, the baby that you were going to have. That will go on for years – it will never stop. Even if we are lucky enough to adopt, we'll never have our own biological child.

I do feel I've grown through the process, which sounds like a really stupid thing to say because who would go through that to grow. It's the hardest thing I've ever had to go through.

Giving up has brought a huge sense of relief. I realised that it had taken over my life and I felt as if I was getting my body, my psyche and my life back.

Since we've stopped, people have said things like, 'That's what you need to do. The minute you stop, it works.' It drives me mad. I feel like shaking them and saying, 'I've got blocked fallopian tubes. It is a physical impossibility.'

The inference is that it's somehow emotional. I did start to feel that I was responsible. The difficult thing is living with the fact that other people are controlling your life when you're going through all this. They're physically taking control of your body, and everything to do with whether or not you're going to have a kid. All you do is provide a womb, and some eggs, and some sperm. In a way, thinking that I could somehow make a difference was part of trying to fight against the feeling that there was nothing I could do. That's why it makes me so mad when people say it's really good we've given up because now I'll get pregnant. I just feel like hitting them.

The hospital we went to had a unit for people who had experienced miscarriage, yet there is no support for childlessness. The private hospital had a counsellor. A friend who had a miscarriage after treatment there told me what the counsellor said to her after the miscarriage: 'Why don't you go out and buy a new nightie?' You've lost the child you've tried for for five years, so what's going to make you feel better? A nightie.

There's all this amazing medical support, and yet, in order to do the medical stuff, emotionally you need the constitution of an ox. There's no emotional support.

Tom: I suppose that's medicine. The whole medical industry is about fixing people. You go there for a cure, so that's all they think about. Infertility treatment is an industry – an industry that's founded on hope. All the talk is about 'We can make this happen.' It's one of the things I found frustrating about the fertility group meetings we went to. It was all about what was the best hospital and how the drugs are working for you – but it's all fantasy, it's all hope which is continually shattered. You are sold this fantasy that you're going to do it, and it's going to work.

Debbie: They said that at the private hospital. They said if it hadn't worked by the third time, they were doing something wrong. The consultant said to us, 'We're looking at take home baby rates here. I want to give you a baby to take home.'

It was like going shopping. I was convinced she was going to give us a baby that we could take home, as if she had some sort of magical power.

Tom: I was desperate to believe it, because I still want a child more than anything else. They sit there full of authority, with facts and figures and knowledge at their fingertips. There's still a part of me that believes that if we went back it could work next time. We've stopped for now, and it's such a relief, but I'm still thinking that in two years' time we may change our minds.

Debbie and Tom have just started going through the first stages of the adoption process, and have had their preliminary assessment meeting.

Debbie: It's the same process as for domestic adoption. You have to have a home study report, and you have to be approved by the adoption panel. Then the overseas bit kicks in. The Home Office have to approve you, and you have to register with the Foreign Office post in the country in which you wish to adopt. Your papers are sent through to the agency in that country, who matches you with a child.

Tom: There's something to pin some hope on to. When you look at the bureaucracy, realistically I can't see a child being in this house for eighteen months minimum. Overseas adoption has its

own set of problems. There's a loss of control. It goes to bureau-
crats on the other side of the world.

Debbie: We saw a social worker from our local authority, and it
was the first positive news we've had. With every hospital
investigation we'd just had more and more bad news, every
treatment had gone wrong – and then in comes this woman and
says, 'Yes, you could be parents.' I wanted to hug her. After four
years she says yes, you could be a parent. That was just great.

KATIE AND MICHAEL'S STORY

'I do hope the woman who donated to us knows . . . We'd
like to feel she knew what she'd done for us . . . and how
absolutely happy we were.'

**Katie is thirty-seven and her husband Michael is thirty-six.
They had unsuccessful fertility treatment before discover-
ing that Katie had been through a premature menopause,
and that they would need to consider using an egg donor.
Their son was born after their first IVF attempt using a
donated egg, and they are now on the waiting list for
another.**

Katie: I was thirty-two when we started trying for a baby. I'd had
mild endometriosis and I thought that was probably why things
weren't working. I went to the GP after six months because of
that, and they referred me very quickly.

I had a laparoscopy and they checked, but the endometriosis
was still only very mild. They said to go away and keep trying
because there was nothing wrong. We were just left to get on
with it for a while.

Michael: I suppose at the beginning it was more of a worry for
Katie than it was for me. I have always been the sort of person
who looks on the bright side. The initial drive to go and see
whether there was a problem came from her. I would probably
have sat still for a bit longer.

Katie: I started to get fed up very quickly because I'd always known I had endometriosis, and I thought there might be a problem. I was eager to get things started, so after another six months in which nothing happened we asked to be referred to a consultant. He didn't do any tests but put me straight on to Clomid, which made me feel diabolical. I think I lasted a month on Clomid, because I couldn't stand it. That was at the local private hospital.

We asked for a referral to another consultant we'd heard about locally, who was more interested in doing all the various tests. He suggested intra-uterine insemination. It was still unexplained infertility.

We did four IUI cycles, none of which worked and all of which he said were perfect. We spent a year doing this because he told us to have a couple of months in between each one. With the last couple, I was ovulating very early and feeling dreadfully ill. Because I was feeling so ill he said he'd do another laparoscopy, and he found the endometriosis had spread. He said we had a choice of treating my endometriosis or going on to IVF. He said it didn't make any difference, but I might feel better if I had treatment for the endometriosis. We decided to push on for IVF.

Michael: We had asked people about where to go, and heard some bad stories about the London clinics: sitting in the corridor, walking in and then bang and out you go again – cattle market stuff. The advice and guidance we received was that you'd get treated better if you went locally, and when you start out in this process you follow the advice you're given.

I was too easily taken in by the funny bow ties and the posh voices. I thought, 'This guy must know what he's about.' It was Katie who thought two and two doesn't make four with this guy – he doesn't make sense.

Katie: By that stage we weren't particularly happy. We were paying an awful lot of money at this private hospital but didn't feel we were being looked at thoroughly. By then we'd read up about all the different hospitals, and we made the decision to go to one in London.

So we went up to London, where they did a blood test and said

I was menopausal. I had been feeling terribly unwell since I was thirty. I'd had lots of different symptoms and been to hospitals, but they kept saying, 'There's nothing wrong with you.' I think that's the part that really upset me so much – that for so long people had said there was nothing wrong, and then to be told the truth. It was so final, knowing that I could never have a child.

I felt devastated, and very angry about not being diagnosed earlier. I'd spent so many years not only feeling unwell but undergoing completely unsuitable fertility treatment. We did the IUI cycles but they didn't do any blood tests. I did urine tests, but apparently there's no value in them at all. The consultant at the local private hospital was telling me to have IVF, and I could have found myself going through that without having any eggs. We were paying them a lot of money – they were more expensive than some of the London clinics.

As soon as I'd found out I went back to the original hospital. They said that there was absolutely nothing wrong, but I had copies of my blood tests which showed the hormone levels. Basically, they'd just misread my results. I was ready to attempt to take legal action, but it would have cost a fortune. We did write to the consultant, and got a very offish reply. In the end I just had to accept that there was nothing I could do. It took me a long, long time to come to terms with that.

I've often asked myself what we could have done, and I think we should have held out to go to a proper infertility clinic. We'd asked to, and we'd been told we didn't need to. A lot of people get their problems solved at a local clinic, but I'd say don't waste too much time there. The main thing is finding out what the problem is, even if you go to a major clinic just for a diagnosis. *Michael*: We'd wasted time and effort, all due to the hospital's laziness. They'd done half the tests – it was the other half that would have pointed to the real reason.

Their process probably fits 80 per cent of the patients they stuff through it, but we were in the other 20 per cent. They would have just carried on taking our money. We'd probably still be there today having more IUIs if we hadn't taken the decision to stop. There must be a lot of people out there who go through fertility treatment and give up believing the treatment hasn't worked, when quite often they will have had incorrect treatment.

Katie: When we went for a second consultation in London they said our only way forward was egg donation, but there was a terrible shortage of egg donors and they didn't know if they could get us one. My first reaction, though, was that I didn't want egg donation anyway. I suppose it was shock. We started looking into adoption, and a year later we'd been approved.

Even so, Katie and Michael decided to go on the waiting list for an egg donor and at least try that route.

Katie: We gave it a lot of thought, and assumed it would be a woman who had completed her family who would donate an egg. The success rate they quoted was 45–47 per cent. The chances are much higher because they're using a fertile woman's egg.

I went to see another consultant who looked after egg donation and asked to go on the list. We had counselling and they took our details – eyes, colouring and height – but said they couldn't always match the donors as well as they'd like because of the shortage. They said I could introduce a friend to be a donor, but I didn't really know anyone I could ask. I think a lot of people do it to help their friends – if you introduce somebody you go to the top of the list.

I definitely think egg donors should be paid expenses and shouldn't be out of pocket in any way, but I'm not so sure about them being paid. I think they've got a lot to think about – about why they're doing it. I'm sure there are a lot of people who know how awful infertility is, and who want to help someone else. It was very important to me that the donor had completed her family. There's no way I'd have eggs from sharing with somebody who was going through IVF. It would be dreadful if it worked for me and not for the person who had donated the eggs.

We had to do an intensive six-week assessment programme during which they build up the lining of the womb and test it.

Normally you do the assessment cycle and then you go straight on to the donation. But they hadn't got a donor available, so after the assessment I was put on to HRT until one became available.

Michael: I haven't told many people about our situation. There's only one colleague at work I've talked to about it – it's not the sort of thing you talk about over a pint. The people I've spoken to were outside the circle of people who understood fertility problems, and they didn't really understand what egg donation was.

Katie: My friends were very good. They'd say they were trying for a baby, telling me rather than keeping it from me. The only time I found very difficult was when I was diagnosed. Then it took me a little while because it was such a final thing.

There's a group called Daisy Chain for people who've had a premature menopause, and when we were waiting I met a lot of people in the same situation. I joined the local Issue group as well as Daisy Chain. Talking about it makes a lot of difference. You know you're not the only one, and the others understand exactly how you feel. People going through IVF have a lot of problems, but with premature menopause you've got different problems – your long-term health and the wait for an egg donor.

At one stage the consultant said, 'Yes, it will be next month,' so we didn't book a holiday. But it didn't turn out to be next month, and everything went on hold for a long time.

Most things in your life you can do something about, but with this you couldn't. I did try. I advertised locally for an egg donor and had one response, but the lady was too old. In the end you had to shut off from it, because there was nothing you could do. I knew that somehow, whether it was through egg donation or adoption, we would manage to have a family. That was the only thing that kept me going.

Michael: When we first talked about egg donation they explained it was a two-year wait, so there were no false hopes. It was just one of those things: take it or leave it.

Katie: Our waiting time was only about a year, which is very short indeed for egg donation. The consultant said it would be after Christmas, and then all of a sudden out of the blue in

October I had a phone call to say she'd got a donor for me, which was absolutely fantastic. I was delighted.

I have a feeling that somebody dropped out along the line and I was fitted in very quickly. I started my drugs the following day, and within two weeks I'd had the embryos put back, so the donor must have started a while back.

Michael: It was something that we did together. I didn't feel outside it. I think I went to the majority of the appointments. From time to time it was quite difficult trying to fit the whole thing in with work.

Katie: You tend to share a donor with somebody else because there is such a shortage, but we were very lucky to have a donor to ourselves, so we had all her eggs. She produced eight, but only three fertilised. Two were good-quality and one was poor, so they put all three back. They normally only put two back, but I think they were sure that the third one was no good. I remember having the embryos put back and wondering what the person was like who had donated them.

Michael: I was there for the embryo transfer. You have to wear the gown and the mask and the hat and the boots. It wasn't overwhelming, but there was a lot to take in. If I ever did it again I'd understand a lot more – I'd be far more receptive to what was going on.

Katie: Originally we'd been told that they'd give us a form with the details of the donor, but we never managed to get that. Apparently the donors are asked if they want to fill in a form and they don't always want to. We don't know anything about the donor, not even her age. Now I'm quite happy about that, but it took me a little while to come to terms with it.

It was a long wait, during which I had injections. I was doing some temping work at the time, and I decided to keep that going. They do a blood test on day 10 and I hadn't even thought about doing a pregnancy test. It didn't even cross my mind, although I know a lot of people do. The day before I went for the blood test I had this dreadful urge to go out and get Chinese for lunch. I've never done that before. I went out and got myself some prawn crackers and sesame toast and ate it, and was violently sick that night. I did wonder whether I was pregnant, because I'm never sick normally. The following morning, when I went up for the blood test, they said it was probably the drugs that had caused me to be sick.

I had the blood test at eight o'clock in the morning and wouldn't get the results until mid-afternoon. It was a hard day. I decided to go to work, and Michael was staying at home so he would be taking the call. The doctor phoned at four to say it was positive.

I was elated. I know some people say they can't believe it, but I think I had a good idea I was pregnant and I could believe it. I had to have extra progesterone for the first three months, and I was on hormone treatment until the placenta took over, after which everything worked naturally. I'm sure that over the nine months of pregnancy I really built up a bond. Even when I had the baby, I still thought about the egg donor a lot, not that it makes any difference to the way I feel about him.

I think people are quite used to the idea of sperm donation, but egg donation is a little bit different, probably because there aren't as many egg donation babies. I've told my friends, but I'm not so keen on telling older people. I understand there's a book on donor insemination babies, so I'm hoping they're going to do a book on egg donor babies. A lot of people know anyway, and most have reacted very well. I think it helps to talk about it.

Michael: I think we've both agreed that we'll tell our son reasonably early in his life. We've spoken to other people who've adopted children, and had a conversation with a friend about how he told his children that they were adopted. If anything, it was easier for him because his wife was never pregnant and there's less to explain. The actual detail of explaining that Katie was pregnant and gave birth to him, but she's not his genetic mother . . . how do you explain that to a young child?

Katie: It's common for doctors not to diagnose a premature menopause. When we were going through the tests it didn't cross my mind, even though I'd been feeling unwell. When I look back I probably had the classic symptoms: I felt sick, nauseous and flushed and there was a change in my personality – a lot of minor things which came on bit by bit. I felt mentally strange, but that wasn't something you could go to the doctor about. I put it down to the fact that we were having problems producing a child.

The premature menopause was absolutely the worst thing that's ever happened to me in two ways: the loss of fertility and the illness. I'm still trying to get sorted out on the HRT tablets, which I've had great problems with. I get diabolical headaches and can't find any tablets which suit me, so it's a real problem. I don't seem able to regain my health, and I just wish I could go back to how I was, to get my health back.

Nevertheless, we have our much longed-for baby. I do hope the woman who donated to us knows. At the time we were told we couldn't make any contact in writing, but I understand now that some couples have made contact with their donors. We'd like to feel she knew what she'd done for us, that I was pregnant and how absolutely happy we were. I do think it's an awful lot for a woman to go through for somebody else.

As soon as we had the baby we thought we'd like to do it again. We asked our GP to write, and we've been on the list a year and a half now. I have no idea how long the wait is. All we know is that it's a lot longer than last time. I don't think it's a very strict list, but I'd imagine we're not top priority – which is fair enough. We're hoping we'll hear some time next year.

CLAIRE AND TONY'S STORY

'We'd gone in happy, pregnant with three children, come out and we were arranging three funerals. It was as simple as that.'

Claire and Tony are both in their mid-thirties. Tony is a builder, and Claire, who used to work as a hairdresser, now looks after their son. Their first IVF attempt was unsuccessful but after their second attempt, using frozen embryos, they discovered Claire was pregnant with triplets. The babies were born prematurely and all three

died within days of their birth. Claire and Tony decided to continue with treatment, and now have a young son.

Tony: We'd been trying for about six months and thought something wasn't quite right. We spoke to other people and they recommended that we see a doctor. We went for an appointment and said we'd been trying for eighteen months, knowing that then he'd say he'd look into our problem.

Claire: My periods had stopped and the doctor prescribed Clomid, which he said would make me ovulate. I was on that for about six months but nothing happened. We went back after the Clomid and they tried to do some post-coital tests, which didn't seem to be very successful. It was a nightmare. I remember leaving the hospital one day and crying.

I had a laparoscopy and they found that my right ovary and tube had been removed when my appendix had been taken out, and the ovary on the left side looked larger than it should have been, because I had endometriosis. That's when the doctor recommended that we go for IVF. We went to a private clinic in 1991 and the consultant was very positive. He gave us the option of treating my endometriosis or going for IVF.

Like many couples Tony and Claire had limited funds, so they chose IVF as the safest option.

Tony: We only had so much money and we had to spend it the best way possible, taking our best chance. One of the fundamental reasons not to have surgery to treat the endometriosis was that if something had gone tragically wrong and annihilated the ovaries there would be no eggs, nothing. So we thought we'd take the IVF route.

Claire: I had all my injections and everything went quite well. Tony did some, a friend who is a doctor did a few, and if I was at the clinic to have a scan they did them there. At that stage I wanted to be given as little information as possible, because that gave me less to worry about. I just thought I have these injections, they get my eggs, put them in and then hopefully we'll have a baby. That was the stumbling block, not getting the eggs.

Tony: Claire had one ovary, but we never for one minute thought that a woman might not actually produce an egg. I thought they give you this drug and then it goes without saying – the only question is how many.

That said, it was a clinic record! Twenty-nine eggs out of one ovary at one go.

Claire: They put me to sleep. I remember waking up and they were saying, 'Bernard Matthews is just lying on the bed, she's got all her eggs out.' They were really nice there, so friendly.

The problem was that, because there wasn't long between egg collection and having the embryos put back in, I was still quite sore. I could have done with another week.

Tony: We were on a tight budget. We knew that this time was going to be our one bite of the cherry, and then we'd have to wait a while. I felt the doctor had had plenty of opportunity to scan Claire – he must have scanned her about twenty-five times. We got into the operating theatre and I thought it would be a simple process – they've got the fertilised eggs, they're going to put this catheter in and put the eggs back in through it. Ten minutes went by and you could see beads of sweat forming on his brow. Then twenty minutes. Finally he said, 'There's going to be a little bit of pain now'. He was tugging and pulling and you could see blood on swabs, and I thought things couldn't be right. It was awful. Then he explained to Claire, 'Unfortunately you've got a kink in your cervix and we can't get the catheter in.'

Claire: They'd only got one egg in. The other two were still in the tube. They said I should come back the next day when they'd give me a general anaesthetic and put the other two in, which they did. I was actually feeling contractions where they'd pulled me about so much.

Tony: Claire had the anaesthetic and they put the other two embryos in. But we both felt it had failed. Sure enough, she started bleeding. It was a disaster.

I wrote the doctor a really snotty letter. I was angry because he didn't see that was our one go – that was all our money gone. I didn't see how he could defend himself and say he hadn't realised Claire had a kink in her cervix.

Claire: I had fifteen embryos in the freezer. Each time we'd get so far and then I'd have to have a cervical dilatation under general anaesthetic before I could have more embryos put in. I had two lots of that before it was called off because they weren't happy. That was really distressing.

I remember one day leaving the clinic as someone was coming in with their twins to show them off. How I got home I don't know. I remember coming in and ringing Tony at work and sobbing down the phone. The pressure and the stress that it puts on you as a couple is unbelievable.

Tony: The big thing for me was the peer pressure. All our friends were having babies, but we didn't tell people about our problems. We obviously didn't spend our money on things like exotic holidays, so they thought we were tucking it all away for a rainy day. But we weren't – we were trying to pursue this infertility thing.

People who have got fertility problems don't know how to deal with them, and people who *haven't* got them certainly don't know how to deal with them, so they're not going to help you out. They don't know how you feel. Infertility and the loss of a child are things that people only talk about once they've been through them.

Next time around they were successful, to their great joy.

Claire: On the next attempt they induced ovulation and then did a Doppler scan to see what the blood flow was like. I had the cervical dilatation. They got three embryos and I didn't look at them this time – I'm very superstitious. They put the embryos in and it took two minutes.

I felt fine, perfectly normal. I was due to go back for my pregnancy test on the Tuesday but I said I'd wait. I told Tony I'd go on the Thursday, my day off. I drove up, had the test and went back home. We were supposed to ring at three-thirty and it was about four-thirty by the time we got back. I was hanging the washing out in the garden when I heard Tony scream.

Tony: I rang up and they said, 'We've been trying to get in touch with you,' and I knew from that moment. I thought, 'Claire's

pregnant.' Even now it makes the hairs on the back of my neck
go up.

They said, 'Are you sitting down? Claire's pregnant.'

I went, 'Yes!' and I threw the phone straight up to the ceiling
and cut them off. It was brilliant.

When they scanned Claire they saw one, then another and
then a third. But the doctor said it was very weak, and if we were
going to tell friends it was more than one we should tell them it
was twins, because that was more than likely the way it was
going to end up.

Claire: He said he wouldn't be surprised if when I came back for
the next scan one had gone. But when we went back it was still
triplets.

I felt awful. I was so full of hormones. I couldn't eat. The only
thing I could drink was Lucozade. My Mum came round one day
and I was trying desperately to be normal. I was in bed with a
quilt over me and she came in and just cried. She said she
thought then that she didn't think I was going to make it – I was
whiter than the sheets.

Tony: That's another criticism of the private IVF system. It was,
'You're pregnant – goodbye.' You're handed over to your local
hospital, and that's where it all started going wrong.

We were shown round the maternity ward and the special
care unit. One of our questions was whether it would be a
caesarean or natural birth. They told us that the last two sets
of triplets delivered there had been vaginal deliveries – no
problems. We were so naive we didn't even realise they'd only
got two incubators – so what about triplets? If you have a
multiple pregnancy you've just got to be in a major teaching
hospital.

Claire: I went in at twenty weeks because I was starting to feel
sick again. The doctor said to me, 'If you can just get to thirty
weeks, you'll stand a good chance,' but things like that don't
sink in. I know you're a bit brain-dead when you're pregnant,
but I couldn't imagine losing the triplets. We thought they
might be a bit premature, but losing them never entered our
heads.

When I was twenty weeks and I stayed in overnight there was a girl in the hospital who had gone into labour at twenty-four weeks, and the baby had died at birth. I can remember seeing people coming in with flowers, but even then that was somebody else.

Tony came in from work one day and this stuff like a mucus plug had come out.

Tony: I told Claire that it looked pretty serious to me. We went to the hospital and I told them what had happened, but the doctor said it would re-form and there was nothing to worry about.

Imagine the scenario. There's a woman with triplets at twenty-four weeks. Should she have been in a hospital with two incubators and no intensive care unit for babies, or should she have been in a large hospital which could cope?

Claire: They said they'd keep me in overnight and I kept saying to them, 'Am I in labour? Am I in labour?', because I knew then that if I was I'd be in trouble.

They said, 'No, you're not in labour. Calm down. We're keeping you in, and remember you're not in labour.'

I remember the midwife saying there was no point in putting a monitor on me because I had three. So they didn't even put a monitor on to see if I was having contractions.

I stayed in there until the Friday. By then I was feeling quite relaxed and thinking that obviously they were right. I said that morning that I'd like to go home for the weekend, and I did.

Then on the Sunday morning I woke up and I had pains coming quite regularly. I thought I was having Braxton Hicks contractions and I went back into hospital. I remember sitting on another girl's bed and we were laughing and joking, but at the same time I was thinking something wasn't quite right. I went and got the nurse, and she was the first person to say she'd put a monitor on me. I was contracting every five minutes. They did an internal and I was five centimetres dilated. I remember bursting into tears and getting hysterical.

Tony: Claire was in full labour and we went to another hospital by ambulance. It was the rush hour, and we had a nurse with us who kept being violently sick. They had a drip to slow the contractions down, but there was nothing to hang it on.

When we got to the hospital, though, everything seemed to go nice and calm. We were in a place that was used to all of this. They examined Claire and the doctor said he could feel one of the babies' heads.

Claire: It had to be a caesarean because they'd have had no chance of surviving a normal birth. The contractions would have crushed their heads.

Tony: They ummed and ahhed for what seemed quite a long time about whether to bother that night or to wait. The consultant was there and Claire was going to deliver in the next six to twelve hours no matter what, so why not have this expert do it as opposed to hanging on for six hours and then having to deal with an emergency? But after the event you do wonder whether the contractions would have stopped if we'd said we'd wait.

They were born, two boys and a girl – Thomas, Connor and Sophie. Thomas was 1lb 11 oz, Sophie was 1lb 7 oz and Connor 1lb 8 oz.

Thomas went to another hospital because ours didn't have enough capacity – they already had somebody there who was expecting quads. Although she wasn't due to deliver for a number of weeks they said she was their priority because she was there. I said we must be the priority because our babies were already born, but they said it didn't work that way.

Claire: Thomas was the best weight. He was lively, he'd cried at birth and he was quite with it, so they said he was the one who could travel.

Tony: I remember being literally on my hands and knees with my arms around this bloke's legs begging him not to send one of them away, but he said, 'There's nothing I can do.' The way he saw it was that we were in a self-inflicted predicament, because they were IVF babies.

Thomas was moved out and we were told that, if everything stabilised over the first seventy hours, things were looking better for survival. No one talked about brain damage and so on – it was just survival. We didn't realise the potential problems even then. We just thought our babies were born early, they would stay in hospital for a long time and then they would come out.

Claire: They died in the order they were born, Sophie first. They came in the middle of the night. I'll never forget it. They turned the lights on, and this lady came in. She said, 'You'd better come down.' I remember saying, 'She's going to be all right?', and she said, 'It would be best if you came down.'

It was strange because I kept saying, 'Ring my husband and get him to come up,' and Tony walked through the door.

Tony: I'd gone home to go to bed, but I couldn't sleep. I didn't sleep at all for the first three or four days after the birth. I walked in, and they said they were going to have to make a decision to turn off the machines.

Claire: Sophie had internal bleeding and had bled so much that she would have been severely disabled. There are stages of bleeding, and a two means cerebral palsy, blindness or deafness. Sophie had a count of four which was the maximum. They like you to make the decision. They take everything off the baby and you get the first chance to hold it.

Then they came up again and said we had to get over to Thomas. I hadn't even seen Thomas. We had to get a cab over there.

Tony: They didn't have an ambulance, so thirty-six hours after being on an operating table Claire had to get into a cab. Thomas had been blessed by a priest, and we weren't even there. He died, and then we came back and Connor died.

We'd gone in happy, pregnant with three children, come out and we were arranging three funerals. It was as simple as that.

Everyone was heartbroken. The doctors involved said it was extremely unusual. Claire was actually twenty-five weeks and three days which, although it was exceptionally early, wasn't unheard of. At twenty-one weeks babies can survive.

Claire: We came out. We had the funerals. Then we just shut the curtains and locked the doors. We couldn't stop crying. I used to do a lot of writing – that used to help me.

You get very angry. People would moan about things and you'd think, 'You don't know how lucky you are.'

We definitely felt after our bereavement that we needed to be very close.

Tony: I changed my career. I was working in structural engineering. I'd always been good with my hands and I used to prepare drawings and plans for other builders. I thought I'd do it myself instead. If I was working for myself and I needed to be with my wife, that's where I was going to be.

You couldn't control the emotion at all, couldn't even mention their names. We got no help from the clinic, no real input, no connection with other people. You're on your own.

The worst scenario is when you're walking around the supermarket doing the shopping, and you've got this woman with about eight kids around her and she's smacking them and swearing, and you think, 'We only want one. What's wrong with us?'

At that point we swore to each other that we would never try IVF or anything like it ever again. We shook hands on that.

Claire and Tony joined a multiple birth association support group for bereaved parents.

Claire: It gave me a chance to go somewhere and cry without making Tony feel really sad. I could cry with total strangers and not feel guilty about it. It was emotionally draining, but I had to go. Also, it was nice to see people who had had the same experience and to know I wasn't some sort of freak.

They're very much: 'We are parents. We've had children.' You need people to see that you are a mother. I remember trying to explain when my sister had a daughter that I desperately needed to take the baby out for a walk. I wanted people to see me with a baby and think, 'She's just had a baby', rather than walk around with nothing. I wanted the recognition. I remember taking her baby to the park and just trying to feel like a mother. Because you *are* a mother. You desperately *feel* like a mother.

Tony: Having triplets is not that unusual any more, but they're nearly all IVF. If you think that to keep a baby in intensive care costs £1,000 a day, to keep triplets is £3,000 a day. Some triplets are born at twenty-eight weeks and stay there until they are term, so that's twelve weeks and more than £250,000 of NHS funds on those triplets.

You'd more than likely find that you could run a whole IVF programme if you only put one embryo in, eradicating many of the problems associated with intensive care. And you could fund the IVF programme as well, because you wouldn't have to spend all that money on those babies that were born and had problems.

The clinic had stuck to their end of the bargain. They had made Claire pregnant. We can't blame them for being over-successful. We know people on IVF who have had two embryos put in and have produced triplets. The one rule of IVF is that there are no rules. Things like this happen. It's quite incredible, really.

Claire and Tony decided that they would try again, using the embryos they still had frozen at the clinic.

Claire: On our third attempt we had two embryos put in. I was convinced I wasn't pregnant. We did a test and Tony said, 'It's positive. You're pregnant.' But I thought it was probably the drugs I was on.

Tony: The euphoria of finding out that Claire was pregnant the second time, with just one baby, was very tainted – we weren't ecstatic. It was the longest nine months of our lives.

We'd put our names down for adoption way before the triplets, and right out of the blue in the middle of an IVF attempt they wrote to us and said we'd been selected to come along and see if we'd be suitable for adopting. One of the criteria was 'Are you having fertility treatment?' We said, 'No, of course not.' During the first meeting Claire was actually at the clinic having the eggs put back in, and I was there on my own. By the third and final one, we'd found out Claire was pregnant.

That was an insight. Let's say you're a responsible adult.

You've pursued a bit of further education, seen a bit of the world. You're twenty-five, twenty-six, you've got no real money behind you but you meet the person you want to spend the rest of your life with . . . You're thirty and you've got enough money, bought a house and you want to start a family. You've got a fertility problem, but it's eighteen months before they'll look into it, so you're thirty-two . . . You have a few attempts at IVF and they don't work . . . You're thirty-five and start to think about adoption, and you're too old. If you work on that basis you'd need to know you've got a fertility problem at about sixteen.

It's only now that you notice posters stating that parents for adopted children are desperately needed, but these are kids with major emotional or psychological problems . . .

We were back at the same hospital. The doctor's advice was to go for an elective caesarean a month early because Claire had already had one caesarean, and if that scar ruptured, as it might during normal labour, we wouldn't only lose the baby, I'd lose my wife.

They scanned her and said the baby was going to be around six or seven pounds, so I thought there was no chance of a problem on that score.

Claire: I was thirty-six weeks. It was a really weird feeling. I was out in the garden, knowing I had to go in that night and have the baby the next day. I felt I could have gone on quite happily and kept saying to Tony, 'I really don't want to have this baby yet.' Even when I was in hospital, I kept thinking we could hang on for a while and perhaps just monitor me for a week or two.

They took me down to the special care unit as a matter of course and showed me round. It was awful.

The next day came, and Tony and our parents and my sister came in. Everyone was being quite relaxed, but I felt so nervous.

Tony: Everyone else seemed quite confident. During that pregnancy we had the anniversary of our loss and the funeral, and it reawakened our guilt that we'd caused all that pain to three babies.

Max popped into the world at 3.42 a.m. on 13 July, and they

took him through to clean him up. You've all got masks on and you're all looking – all you've got is eye contact and eye movement. The eyes are pretty expressive, and as I looked at the doctor and the nurse I could see they were having a conversation with their eyes. I asked what the problem was, and they said, 'It's this thing. It can't be working. It measures the oxygen in the baby's blood and it's coming up at 72. That must be wrong because it's got to be over 90.'

They did it again and it was 100, and then they did it one more time and it was 68. Then they looked at his chest and it was dipping. They said they weren't going to take the baby back to Claire but to the special care unit. Everything was going through my head and I thought, 'We're going to lose him. There's no doubt about it. We're going to lose him.'

Max was taken to the unit by ambulance, taking a really slow, long route because they didn't want to bump the baby around. I was already there when he appeared. They did a quick check on him and looked at the X-ray, which they described as worse than useless. The local hospital hadn't sent any of our notes because they said the photocopier was broken and they couldn't release the original documents. The doctor there had put the ventilator pipe in so deep that he'd scratched one of Max's lungs, and they had cut his cord too short so they couldn't take blood. They'd seriously messed up.

Claire: If you give birth naturally babies' lungs get pushed about because of the contractions and they start to breathe. Because Max had been born by caesarean and hadn't been given any stress his lungs were still full of fluid, and because he'd taken a deep breath to cry and filled them with air it was as if he was drowning.

He was in intensive care for about twenty-four hours and then he was in special care. We didn't have him for nine days. There was absolutely no question that he was going to die as far as they were concerned, but for us . . . From that day to this he's been fine.

We did get a lovely bouquet of flowers from the IVF clinic. We took him up to show them and they were lovely. That was the icing on the cake. Taking Max up there and seeing people in the waiting room looking at me as I had looked at that woman with twins. It was like going full circle.

Claire and Tony are hoping to have another child. They had another unsuccessful IVF attempt and then decided to go ahead with surgery for Claire's endometriosis. The operation went well, and their consultant is optimistic that it may be possible for Claire to conceive without further medical help.

JANE AND MARK'S STORY

'When they hear I've had two natural pregnancies, every doctor says, "Come to me, I can do it." They think they can do it, but they can't.'

Jane and Mark are both teachers. They have had IVF treatment over a period of ten years but without success. They've been to seven clinics, and have had fourteen full IVF cycles and a number of frozen embryo transfers. During this time Jane has had two natural pregnancies, but both were ectopic. Jane is now forty and Mark forty-seven. They have decided not to have any more treatment.

Jane: When we first decided to start a family, I got pregnant the first cycle. But I had an ectopic pregnancy. We knew then that there might be a problem, because I only had one tube left. When I hadn't got pregnant within a year we were already starting to think about possible problems and infertility, so it didn't come out of the blue. We went on the IVF waiting list, and it was going to be a two-year wait.
Mark: This was for a research programme where you were paying a contribution – nothing like the cost of a private IVF attempt. While we were waiting to get to the top of the list to go on the programme we decided we'd pay for private treatment,

partly so we could time it to take place in the long school summer holidays.

Jane: That first year we couldn't afford both to pay and have a holiday anyway. We had to go to a place which could fit us in over the holidays, and ended up not thinking too hard about where we went. We got a list of clinics which did IVF, and there weren't that many to choose from. I did it by ringing them up and seeing if they sounded nice and helpful on the phone. We didn't ask the right sort of questions – about success rates and whether they had a freezer. This was before they set up the Human Fertilisation and Embryology Authority, and we didn't even have the basic information that bigger centres had higher success rates. So we ended up going to a very small programme in a new set-up with no freezer.

Jane and Mark started their first treatment cycle that summer.

Jane: I remember getting really elated at every scan I had when they said, 'Oh, I can see six follicles,' or despondent when they told me, 'I can only see three.' I now know that what they see on the scans bears very little relation to how many eggs there are. But no one ever tells you that. So long as the follicles are developing, that's all you need to worry about.

Mark: Once we were into it we got really tied up with the successes that came along the way, like the number of eggs that were collected successfully; then the next hurdle we got over – that there had been fertilised eggs; and then that the eggs were put back. Our expectations rose as we went through it.

Jane: It cost between £1,000 and £2,000, and my mother gave us the money. That was something I would never do again. I met another woman who was in the same boat – she'd let her family give her the money and she said she felt she was letting them down. I certainly did.

We had one more private attempt while we were still waiting to come to the top of the list for the research. We went to another hospital which was a bigger, more professional, more successful outfit. We were kicking ourselves that we hadn't gone there the first time. I really thought it was going to work that time. We had a good crop of eggs and put some in the freezer as well, but it didn't work. I was devastated, because by then I felt it was my turn for it to work. That was the worst. We would have gone back there – we liked them and we liked the set-up. But by then we'd come up on the research list.

They told us right from the beginning that we would only get three chances on the research programme. We said that was OK, because if it hadn't worked by then we wouldn't want to do it any more. Famous last words . . .

Mark: The only IVF they did there was their research programme. I think they were using people to further their own research: trying to understand the different stages of IVF and to get better at the whole process. We were grateful to be on the programme, and that we were paying £400 instead of more than £1,000. Because of that situation we probably didn't question them or push them nearly as much as we should have done, and at one point we realised they were taking some eggs off.

Jane: I was trying to track back after an egg collection. I think I had had eighteen collected, and I wanted to know exactly how many of them had fertilised. They said, 'Of course, we only put twelve of your eggs with your husband's sperm because the others are part of our research programme.'

Jane and Mark continued their treatment on the pro-gramme, with some of Jane's eggs being used for research each time.

Mark: There were times there when I felt we were part of a process that we had no control over. We'd gone into a tunnel which we were just being moved along. When we did try to ask questions there was one doctor who was particularly unhelpful and almost evasive.

Jane: I remember an incident when I was having some embryos put back. The doctor had put the catheter through my cervix and then asked me, 'Is it in now?' I said didn't know, and he said,

'Can't you feel it?' I said, 'I can feel that you're doing something. Don't you know?' I just didn't have any confidence in them. I told Mark I didn't even know if the embryos had gone back in the right place. With increasing disillusionment we started to think that it wasn't the IVF that wasn't working – it was just that they weren't doing it properly.

Mark: Jane saw some statistics that showed your chances in relation to the number of attempts you did, and we came to believe that statistically it would happen. The more times we did it, the more likely it would eventually become our turn. I think probably the second, third and fourth attempts when it still wasn't working were the most difficult.

Jane: The first few times I had a general anaesthetic for the egg collection, but at that hospital they could only get theatre time for a general anaesthetic on a Tuesday. Once I was ready on another day, so I had to have pethidine instead. Every time I've had collection under local anaesthetic I've found it very painful, and I have a good pain threshold. I put up with the injections and all the rest of it better than most people, but that I found excruciating. If I have a choice I always have a general anaesthetic. For the last four or five years no one has even suggested that I should have egg collection carried out under local anaesthetic. And if they had suggested it I'd have said no, because I know it isn't for me.

Mark: On the occasions I've been there I've found it very difficult to sit and see her flinching and crying, obviously in pain, when I can't do anything about it. She'd be saying, 'Tell them to give me some more stuff, tell them to give me more.'

There was one collection that was very painful, and the doctor got angry with her after a while because she was flinching so much.

None of their attempts on the programme worked, and Jane and Mark started looking at other clinics.

Jane: I had a friend who was at a teaching hospital and had twins from IVF. She was very active in the patient support group there, and kept telling me I ought to go there – they were wonderful and would sort me out.

I told Mark we had to give them one try at least – we couldn't give up the idea of having children just because we happened to have gone to the wrong place. So we transferred there.

I was very encouraged when we got there, because the first thing the doctor asked was whether anyone had looked at the tube I'd still got left. When I said no he said he'd send me to a brilliant woman who would do a test called a hysterosalpingogram, where they put dye through to see if the passage is clear. He said putting the dye through sometimes helped to clear a blockage, and even if that didn't work she had a new technique that enabled her to open up blocked tubes gently. I went to see her, and she said the tube looked good. It wasn't long after that that I got pregnant again naturally through that tube. I'm sure that putting the dye through did help, but unfortunately that pregnancy was ectopic as well.

I knew on a Sunday I was pregnant, and I phoned the hospital and asked for an early scan. They told me to come on the Thursday, because there was no point in coming too soon. I'd already had some back pain and on the Thursday the doctor said she couldn't see a pregnancy, but it was very early and that didn't necessarily mean it was ectopic. She asked me to make another appointment for eight weeks, when they would know for sure.

By the time I got back to work that afternoon, I'd got all the pains and I knew. I went to the hospital's casualty department and said I was having an ectopic pregnancy. They were brilliant because by then I'd already done IVF several times, and they knew this was what they call a 'precious baby'. They admitted me but then all the pains went away, so they said I could return home and go to the clinic on Monday.

At the clinic the doctor, a senior registrar, said, 'There it is! I can see it in the womb. It's not ectopic. You're fine. Off you go home.' While I was waiting for Mark to come and get me I started to bleed, so they told me to rest in bed with my feet up in the air. I did it for a week, only getting out of bed to go to the toilet, and hoping and praying and wishing and wondering and checking all the time. I lost so much blood I assumed it was a miscarriage.

I had an appointment to see the first woman for another scan. I told her I'd been bleeding all week. She scanned and scanned and scanned, and was getting increasingly concerned. She thought it was ectopic, but I said the other doctor had seen it in my womb. She had a row with him on the phone. They admitted me, and she was right and he was wrong. It was ectopic and they operated that night. There was a photograph of what he'd seen in my womb, and they said it was a pseudo embryonic sac. I think it must sometimes happen.

So that was my second ectopic. I had got no tubes at all now, so it was IVF or nothing. It was almost a relief to lose the second tube because then it wasn't a monthly disappointment, only an every-time-I-had-treatment disappointment.

By then we were going to the teaching hospital, and we liked them very much there. They were nice people, and gave us a good service.

Mark: They were running it on a shoestring. The facilities weren't anything like as good as at the private hospitals, but the people who were running it compensated for that.

Jane: They sometimes kept you waiting for hours and hours, but when we did make appointments to see the consultant to discuss things there was so much time given, no sense of being rushed or pushing you out – it was very human, caring and supportive. They put a lot of effort into making things as friendly as possible for people, and that makes you feel better.

The treatment was different. The only examination room was also the operating theatre, and you'd go in in your outside clothes. I had embryos put back in while I was wearing my outside clothes. They'd say, 'Right, OK, you're done. Off you go,' and you'd pull your knickers back on and walk down the corridor. At other places Mark has had to get into full surgical regalia, and I have had to be wheeled in on a trolley by porters down the corridor just to have my embryos put back in.

Jane and Mark developed strategies to deal with treatment as they went through more IVF cycles.

Jane: We timed the very first one, when we didn't know what to expect, for the summer holidays, and we were going nearly every day for injections and scans. For the second one I took the whole month off work, because I said it was going to be so stressful. Actually it wasn't a good idea, because I sat around and worried. From then on I never took the whole time off. I fitted it around my job, and certainly for the last few times I just had to say I might be ten or fifteen minutes late for work.

Mark: Whether you've been at home or at work, the other issue while this is going on is not telling anybody. That's always been a problem: balancing going to your appointments if you're at work and not wanting people to know where you're going.

Jane: We simply couldn't have managed if Mark hadn't given me the injections. I couldn't have continued going to work if I'd needed injections done by a medical professional every day. It makes a huge difference to coping with a treatment cycle, particularly for that last injection which you have to have at midnight or two o'clock in the morning.

Mark: It was such a strain having to find other people to give the injections that I realised I had to do it. To start with I would push very slowly and gently, and she'd be in agony. I'm amazed that she put up with the bruises and bleeding. It's very easy now. It really is like throwing a dart at her backside. I still don't enjoy it, but now it's not a problem.

Jane: I do the Buserelin by injection as well – that's with tiny little needles which are subcutaneous. I prefer it because I only have to do it twice a day instead of sniffing every four hours.

Mark: We told very few people in the early days. While we were on the first attempt we had friends staying, and we had to disappear mysteriously to have the embryos put back. We told them some sort of lie about having to go and see someone. I remember telling them the truth when it was over – when it hadn't worked. At the time it must have seemed very strange, but there was no way we would have considered telling them.

Jane didn't want people to know something quite so intimate about us. There were times when I did tell people and she would get very upset.

Jane: In the first year or two I didn't want them to feel sorry for me. I didn't want them to know there was a problem, because I felt a failure. Although my brain knows it's not my fault, my heart still says I have failed. I'm sure this is true for lots of women in the same situation. I know it's not true, and I know it's illogical, but a woman who can have children seems a better woman in some way than I am.

Another reason I didn't talk to my friends very much about it was that I didn't want to break down and cry. I think that's something almost above and beyond the call of friendship. I know in a way it's not and I don't mind if my friends cry over me, but I didn't want to do that to them. If we'd gone out in the evening for a drink or something, I thought it wouldn't have been fair of me to burst into tears all over them.

We've told people the principles. We don't make a secret of the fact that we have IVF treatment, but we don't say we're doing it this week, or this month, because we don't want people to get involved in the timings. Then we don't have to tell them when it hasn't worked.

Mark: One thing that became obvious was how little people know about it. Some were anxious to know, but mostly we met ignorance. Perhaps I shouldn't have expected them to know, but I was surprised at how little people understood about what IVF involved. They'd ask some fairly clumsy questions.

Jane: I grew very concerned about Mark, because I wasn't talking to my friends and so I wasn't sharing it with anyone except him. I was leaning too much on him, crying every night and waking him up.

Early on I wasn't very proud of some of my feelings. When friends announced their pregnancies, I would come home and sob and sob and sob. I was able to put a good face on it and offer congratulations, but at the time it hurt. Now it doesn't bother me when people are pregnant because I'm almost past that stage and out the other side. I had heard of other women whose friends were frightened to tell them they were pregnant, and I never wanted it to be like that.

After their fourth unsuccessful attempt at the teaching hospital, they started to look around again. Jane wanted to try another consultant to see whether he might be able to help them before deciding to give up on IVF.

Jane: Although we liked the teaching hospital very much we decided in the end that we needed a more individually tailored programme, since I clearly wasn't a straightforward case. Given the numbers they were dealing with, that hospital had to make things pretty streamlined.

The new consultant said, just like they all had, 'No problem. The fact that it hasn't worked at these other places doesn't make any difference at all. It doesn't mean it won't work here. We can make it work for you.'

Mark: There was a surprising amount of near-animosity – putting other institutions down. We were encouraged to think that we were now in better hands, and I was surprised at his attitude.

Jane: We waited at least two hours to see him. We had an eight o'clock appointment and he arrived in the building at quarter to ten. He asked where we'd been before, and when we told him he said, 'Huh, two of the worst success rates in the country.' He should have known what we had invested in terms of time and energy and money in those attempts at other places. I felt it was unforgivable to dismiss it like that.

Jane and Mark went ahead with treatment under the new consultant, but after four more unsuccessful attempts they decided to try a new tack.

Jane: Our final fling was donor eggs. A friend of mine who had had a premature menopause went to see this man in the Midlands. His success rate for women like her is 66 per cent, which is fantastic. But for people with my problem it's only the same as the normal IVF success rate.

I had some qualms about donor eggs that I'd never had about normal IVF, but never enough to make me consider not doing it. I think it's a fantastic thing that women do for each other. They've got a very good set-up at that hospital. They advertise locally, and they treat their donors exceptionally well.

Jane and Mark had one attempt using fresh eggs and two using frozen embryos from their donor. None were successful, and they have decided that they will not pursue any further treatment.

Mark: The desire to be a parent is much stronger in Jane than it is in me. In a sense that has helped, because when it hasn't worked there's only one set of grief to deal with. For my part I would have given up IVF a long time ago. I wanted to come out of the tunnel. I'd had enough, and I didn't want to go into another one which was about adoption. I'm a bit older than Jane, and the older I've got the less happy I've been about a child coming into our lives like that.

Jane: Mark said right from the beginning he wasn't interested in adoption. Even I would only ever have considered adopting a baby, and babies don't come up very often. So I knew it was a long, long chance.

We've both felt that being a parent is a difficult enough job anyway. To be a parent of an adopted child is just phenomenally difficult with all those extra complications.

Mark: Jane thought about adopting from abroad, but we didn't get into it because of all the horror stories. In all of this – and it's taken a long time – there's no stone that's not been turned over, and there have been times when I've been the brake on Jane's enthusiasm.

As soon as one treatment cycle finished, she was planning the next one. In a sense that was the way in which we didn't have to come to terms with it, because we were going straight on to the next one. It's this thing about knowing that you're doing something, that you're not just sitting there accepting it.

We've done everything. We've cooked up Chinese herbs and drunk horrible things. We've spent hundreds of pounds on vitamins and mineral supplements. We've had allergy tests, zinc tests, hypnotism. We'd do anything and everything. It's nice that we can laugh about them, but we should have known better.

I would have finished some time ago. Jane knew that. But I've never said we weren't going to do it any more. It's something that she had to come to terms with. Through doing all this she's achieved that, whereas if I'd forced the issue and we'd stopped three or four years ago with some avenues still unexplored, we'd have been in a very different situation now.

Jane: I think we've been very lucky because we have money, and we have jobs that we enjoy. Certainly for the last few years we've been able not to let it dominate our lives. There was a time at the very beginning when it was taking every waking moment, and I was resentful that it was taking so much money as well. I remember saying to Mark that one of the pluses of not having children was that we were meant to have enough money for nice holidays and clothes and a house – but we couldn't do that because every spare penny was going on IVF. That really was a Catch 22. There must be millions of people out there for whom the money is a much bigger factor. We resist any attempt to work out how many thousands of pounds we've spent on it.

Mark: Because we both have good jobs and chose to put our money into IVF, we've done it a number of times. But perhaps if we'd been less well off we'd have made the decision to stop a lot sooner. The circumstances would have been different. You can't draw parallels with other people. We had the money and that's what we chose to do with it. People who haven't got the money haven't got the choice, and so perhaps come to terms with their infertility a lot quicker than we did.

Jane: It's terribly easy to stop going for a promotion, to stop planning to go to college or to go on holiday, in case you get pregnant. It's very important not to put it off, because the treatment might not work. Having a satisfying job is what's kept me sane through all of this. It's really very important, because otherwise your whole life is on hold.

There is a very small group of women like me for whom IVF still hasn't worked, even with the top kind of treatment and having done it enough times. Given that I have always produced enough eggs and the eggs always fertilised, it's extremely unusual that it hasn't worked. When they hear I've had two natural pregnancies, every doctor says, 'Come to me, I can do it.' They think they can do it, but they can't.

I have decided there's something wrong with the womb – nothing visible. It must be some minor biochemical thing, and in twenty or thirty years they'll find out what it is. What worried me all the way along is that we might stop and then they would discover it.

Mark: One of the things we've talked about is sex education at school, which is all about not getting pregnant. It's never about the not so small proportion of people who have difficulty conceiving and who never will. The expectation that you will be a mother is very much still there. Even when you've reached the point of doing IVF there's still the expectation that it will work for you.

Jane: Maybe it's to do with our generation, but there's nothing in my life that I've ever wanted that I haven't been able to get by studying, by saving, by waiting, by working. This is the first thing that, however much effort and time I give, I can't get. I would do anything. If I could swim around the world and get a baby I would . . .

You still hear women who are getting married or setting up home with someone saying, 'We're going to do this and this and this and then we've going to start a family,' or 'We're going to wait one year and then we're going to have a baby.' Never with a question mark or 'If we're lucky' or 'God willing' . . . The confidence is incredible. Yet all those women must know somebody it didn't work for.

If we were doing it again, we'd miss out the first one and we'd miss out the research stuff. We were silly in our first choice of hospital because we hadn't found out enough about it, and we were silly not asking more questions about the research programme. But I wouldn't do anything else different. I'm glad I've done everything, and I'm sure I can accept the fact that I'm never going to be a mother knowing that I did absolutely everything I could have done.

POLLY AND MARCUS'S STORY

'I think it's a shame that because we have this technology
you're forced to get on the bandwagon. You don't really
have a choice.'

**Polly manages a day care centre and her husband Marcus
is an artist. Their first attempt at IVF was unsuccessful, and
they decided they would have one more treatment cycle
before trying to adopt a child. After starting the second
cycle Polly discovered she had conceived naturally, but
doctors feared the drugs she had taken meant the baby
might not survive.**

Polly: I had always wanted children, right back to years and years
ago. I met Marcus and we chose to get married because we were
thinking of having kids. For the first six months it was better if
we didn't have a baby, so there was no problem. After that I
started getting edgy.

I remember people saying that you didn't need to worry for up
to two years. Marcus was very laid back about it, but I was
thinking that once we got to two years I'd be allowed to
investigate it. I was very keen to find out answers, to know
what I was dealing with, whereas Marcus felt I was being over
the top. So I had to wait until he was ready to look into it.

Then we met another couple who were having problems
conceiving. They'd already got so far down the line with all
the tests they'd had. That justified it.

Marcus: Polly was starting to get concerned, but I thought she
was being a bit neurotic. I have the advantage of not having the
biological pressure, so I could be objective for the pair of us. I
always thought it would happen at some point, though I realised
that was a luxury I could afford but Polly couldn't. She kept
saying we should think about treatment, but it was only about
then that I felt ready to go to the doctor for some kind of
consultation. I had always had lumpy sperm and, because I'd

never got anyone pregnant and I had been in a relationship where I hadn't used contraception, I thought there might possibly be something wrong.

Polly: The doctor's advice was to go on holiday and relax, which we did. It didn't help at all. Then we did a lot of dancing around looking at clinics – probably because we didn't want to jump into the whole thing. What was so depressing was the idea that you had to become a hospital person, a regular clinic attender. I really didn't want to, and felt quite emotional about it.

Marcus: We did the sperm test first, and the motility turned out to be low. I went to the local hospital to see the specialist, which was terrible. They just asked for a sample and that was that. I had to go to the pathology department and get a sample bottle. There were two secretaries in the room where you take the sample. I said, 'Have you got a toilet?', and one said, 'There's one there.' It had saloon doors, so people could see the top of your head and your feet.

It took me hours to find a better toilet to do the sample in. I had to keep going to different floors, and even then it was just a regular one with gaps at the bottom of the door. I think they must have a policy in hospitals of having toilet doors with a gap at the bottom. There was some guy shuffling and coughing outside, and I just had to wait for him to go.

The first recommendation made to Polly and Marcus was to lead a healthier lifestyle.

Polly: We both smoked marijuana and drank quite a lot, and were told that these two things could affect fertility. Marcus spelled out to the doctor all our sins that I had no intention of telling anybody, which was naive of me because people's lifestyle is so often their problem.

We were hopeful that three months of clean living could solve it. It was really hard. Our evenings were now very different – a great culture shock. We worked on the lifestyle, and it did improve motility but only to just below borderline.

At this stage they decided to take the plunge and go for IVF.

Polly: That's when I waded into IVF. The life we live today makes you very conscious of time running out, and although I dreaded being part of the IVF process I didn't want to contemplate leaving anything to nature. Marcus still did, but to me that was just putting it off. People grieve about not having a baby, but I grieved about not having a natural baby. I remember thinking how sad to have to have someone conceiving our child for us, when it should be born of sex and love.

Marcus: I was pleasantly surprised by how quickly the wheels get into motion. I didn't like the idea of IVF at first, but I knew enough about it to be aware there were no strange effects. You can see by looking at the process that it's all fairly straightforward.

It's quite amazing to have that kind of control. The mystery about conception is that it involves a lot of luck and surprise. To be active in that, to decide when to take the drugs, when the sperm is put in . . . given the odds, you can predict fairly well when you're going to be pregnant. I don't think there's much else like it in life.

I'm glad to have been involved in the evolution of human reproduction, the evolution of fertility. I began to get a holistic view, rather than seeing the technology as an alien thing. The way fertility technology is advancing is becoming part of our fertility – it's not separate.

Polly: I felt I wanted to get to the end of it. I was a complete pessimist, so I found it a comfort to look at the worst case scenario. I quickly became aware that what I was really focussing on was wanting to be a mother, not necessarily mothering my own child. I suspected the quicker I got through IVF, the quicker I could move on to something else like adoption.

I was very aware of what a complete and whole person I would be when I became a mother. I was losing great chunks of myself, and I knew that once I did become a mother I'd be me again. I was keen to get on with it and be complete again. Men are going through it all, but they won't admit it. There was a great emotional difference between the way Marcus and I took it. We had totally opposing views on what my upset was all about.

Whenever I've got anything going on in my life I tell everyone. There's not much they can gossip about if they know it all from you anyway. And I wasn't ashamed of it, although you do end up feeling a bit ashamed when everyone's pumping out kid after kid. At the time I was quite determined that I shouldn't have to be ashamed of infertility, so why should I have to keep it quiet?
Marcus: The first thing people think is that you're impotent. They confuse the whole thing. They think you can't have sex or get an erection. There's a lot of harrumphing and coughing, not really wanting to know too much about it but being sensitive. Then you'd say, 'Look, it's all right. I have sperm. It's just that they don't work that well.' I had to say that line so many times.
Polly: People could never understand how terrible it was. They could never say the right thing. They really didn't have a hope of getting it right. The classic is when you tell them you can't have kids and they say, 'Oh, you know we only had to look at each other and out popped six – I just glanced at her and she was pregnant.' Somehow, even though they've proved their case in flesh and blood, they still want to shoot you down with their almighty sperm.

People did get it wrong a lot. Lots of them feel free to comment, and then suddenly you've got no rights if you've been fool enough to let it out of the bag. I thought these things are known to be sacred, but they're not.
Marcus: Some of my male friends were incredibly brutal with their jokes: 'Oh, we're going to buy you a pair of underpants with a skull on the front' – that kind of thing. Yet other friends were just very delicately enquiring and incredibly sensitive.
Polly: You have no idea of what you're going to go through – you don't know what the reality is going to be like at all. I was quite excited, but a bit gobsmacked. You still sort of wonder if this is your world, if this is really you, but it's all mixed up with eager anticipation that you're going to have a baby, and that this is all going to stop.

I knew there was a gun to do the injections, so I wasn't so frightened of that. I could do them myself, but I liked the idea of him doing it for me and being involved, which was quite nice for him.

Marcus: I didn't like giving those injections because they hurt, but I still felt it was important for me to be involved. It was our thing, and that was the agreement between us. I might have left Polly to it a few times, but we always went to the hospital together.

Polly: The one thing the hospital made a mistake about was that they always used to call me alone in to the appointment. I always thought that was wrong, because it concerned both of us. It was always both of us there. Marcus was quite offended by that.

After believing that the problem was down to Marcus, Polly was surprised to discover that her own fertility might be impaired too.

Polly: The first thing they did was scan me, which revealed that I had polycystic ovaries which they said could cause fertility problems for women. I'd thought all of me was wrapped up – I thought the laparoscopy and everything had told them all they needed to know. The last thing I'd expected right at the stage of doing IVF was the shock news that I might be the cause of this infertility. You feel so safe in the hands of all these professionals, but you begin to realise more and more that you're not. They're just investigating nature, and really the most slippery part of nature, which is quite a tricky thing to do. They can't give any promises or guarantees, and they can't remember to tell you everything that might pop up, so you do get some shocks along the way.

I remember feeling a bit like Marcus must have done, until they told me that because I had regular periods my condition wasn't affecting my fertility. But it did mean we had to start the process tentatively on lower doses of drugs, and that we'd probably have to increase them, which we did. We were told that hyperstimulation would mean the process would have to be stopped, which seems like the worst thing in the world because it's stopping it before it's begun, and once it's begun you feel you're on the way to having a baby.

Because I was on a low dosage of drugs my eggs weren't developing very quickly. But you want results. What was frightening all the way through the process was just how much could go wrong, and how much could mean stopping and calling it a day. You think, having taken a deep breath and gone for IVF, that should be that. But no, there are still just a million hurdles along the way.

Marcus: I felt guilty, because it would seem that the problem was mine and yet all the messing around was going to be done to Polly. The one thing that upset me more than anything else was the fact that she had to take drugs to over-ride her hormonal system. But because she was willing to do it, she told me not to worry about it.

Polly: When I was having my eggs collected I felt really special. I was often aware of the other women in the clinic, and I was thinking I'd got to the grown-up bit.

We went into a room where there was a bed with stirrupy contraptions which looked sadly like everything you've been brought up to think of as a birth bed. The nurse put on some gentle pipe music, which I really hadn't expected. That was quite sweet, actually. It's funny how silly little details like that make you feel a bit special. I got on to the thing and hoisted my legs up. I had the nurse on the right and Marcus on the left, and the doctors explained that they stick something through the ovaries and suck out the fluid. It travels down some hose straight into the analysis room, and they tell you whether there's an egg because there isn't always one in every little pocket that they suck out. You go through terrible agony with a needle stuck through your ovaries – they are telling you to relax but your body is instinctively pulling away from it. I was looking forward to the drugs and felt quite nice and woozy, but they weren't very good painkillers. I'm possibly quite weedy about pain, but it really hurt.

Then you get, 'Yes, it's an egg, it's an egg.' It's a bit like your version of 'It's a boy' or 'It's a girl', but it's just a load of eggs. I remember crying a bit because it suddenly struck me that there I was with Marcus mopping my brow, and the nurse saying, 'It's OK, it won't be long.' It was exactly the scene you picture with birth, though I was giving birth to five microscopic eggs.

It's all a bit sad. It's done, and you're wondering whether or not you're going to have a child now. All the glory leading up to it, and they've just got a few silly eggs in a dish. You're going off, having had this horrible thing done to you, and maybe the bubble's about to burst.

Marcus: It was terrifying waiting to find out whether the eggs had fertilised. That really was a very tense time. I can't think of any equivalent other than waiting for the result of some test or biopsy, but this is not of that nature. It was very strange, very emotional. It was almost like having a baby when you found out they'd actually fertilised. You felt very emotional about it.

Polly: There's twenty-four hours between taking the eggs and being told whether they've fertilised or not. In the morning when I woke up Marcus and I were sadly calm, not talking much, quite mellow and subdued. I was running a bath and I didn't know if I'd heard the phone ring or not. Then Marcus came in and gave me a cuddle and said we'd got two embryos, and we both burst into tears. The relief just to know that we had made a cocktail at all, even if it didn't last long, was so lovely.

We always had a row after going to the hospital, and one of our worst took place after they were put back, which you'd have thought would be a really romantic time. It was sweet to think your babies are put back in you. It was nice to hear that they were all good-quality eggs, even though there weren't very many of them. Everything was grade A at that stage – not that that means anything, but you can't help scoring points anywhere you can at that stage.

The waiting was horrid. You don't know whether they're settling in or not, or whether they're alive or have died. You were wanting to tell everybody you've got something there, that something's happening, but there might just be a period at the end of it.

I was always saying I wasn't pregnant, and everybody thinks

you're being a pessimist and killing your own child with your
negativity. In reality you're staying sane and preparing for the
worst. Your secret hope inside is always enough to keep it alive if
it's going to live.

Marcus: Polly got some bleeding. It wasn't a full period so we
didn't know what that was supposed to mean.

We had mixed feelings when we found out it hadn't worked.
It did mean that we could relax, do something about the tension
that had built up and assess the situation.

For the first time I became active in terms of deciding what we
should do. We had saved enough money for another try, but I
insisted we should go on holiday. I was thinking that if it failed
the second time the pressures would hit hard, and we'd really
need to be in a position to do something active about the
alternatives, to think about adoption.

I persuaded Polly that we should take advantage of the fact
that it hadn't worked. We should do all the cliches, spend the
money and not be too precious about it, indulge in a holiday
before we started a second time, and find an alternative which
was really to cushion the blow should it not work – that was to
adopt from Thailand.

**Polly and Marcus spent a three-week holiday in Thailand
and made use of the opportunity to find out about overseas
adoption, visiting orphanages and meeting the social
workers who would be involved.**

Polly: I was worried whether I would feel proud of an adopted
child. I knew that inside I would love it, but I didn't want to be
like I have been with IVF – being brave. I wanted my experience
of motherhood to be entirely proud, because I've had to be brave
so much in the last few years when other people have got
pregnant and had kids and families.

I sat in the airport coming back and was so thrilled at the idea
of a Thai baby that I really thought at that stage I wanted one
more than my own. It did confirm that I could thoroughly love it
and be really proud to show off my baby. That felt good.

I'd told myself that we would adopt, and that moment was getting nearer because of visiting the orphanages and so on. I was perfectly happy with that prospect. I think I had got over my bereavement and was coming out the other side of grieving. I was beginning to accept fully that I would never have my own child. It was my first big lesson in life.

I had known that what I wanted was motherhood, and I did start to believe that one day, even if it were in another six years, a baby would come. But what I didn't want was another six years of not being a mother, not being in that world of people taking kids to school and fussing about kids, having to think about responsibility – I wanted all that. Motherhood with adoption would have given me that, and I think made me relaxed enough. It's a disgusting fact that I did fall pregnant when I was really relaxed.

Polly and Marcus started their next IVF attempt when they got back from Thailand, without any idea that Polly might be pregnant.

Polly: I wanted to wrap everything up, have a further IVF, move on to adoption and get going. I didn't want delays. I was gladly sniffing again, getting out my little bottle, hoping the whole world could see it going up my nose and wonder about it. I was quite pleased to be doing it again.

Marcus: I had an intuition that she was pregnant, that we might just get in there at the last minute. Her period should have come – she was a day late. She'd started the treatment, and I was thinking that she ought to discover quickly if she was pregnant because of the drugs, whereas she was quite pessimistic about it – I think she didn't want to taste the disappointment again.

Polly: I was due to have my period on the Monday, and it was four days late. You start sniffing a week before your period is due, and it can be delayed because the hormones screw up. I phoned the nurse just in time before the clinic shut on Friday, and when I asked her if I should do a pregnancy test she said yes.

I had a kit left over from when the last IVF failed. I used it and it was positive.

I was really shocked. I phoned the nurse again and told her. I was sure it meant that I had got the wrong pregnancy kit to go with the drugs that I was sniffing, that the drugs had affected my urine and that had I bought the right test it would be normal. But she said, 'Oh God, Polly, that means you're pregnant.' She didn't sound too happy, and asked if I wanted to know the facts: only 50 per cent of these babies survive.

I immediately assumed mine was not going to live, and felt upset that it had ruined my IVF. So I asked her what would happen if I bled, and when I could do IVF again. She said I'd have to wait two or three months, which for me was the worst case scenario. I had no faith in the pregnancy living, even though I wanted it to, and I was angry that all my plans had been put back, so asked her whether, if I bled that night, I could continue sniffing. She must have thought I was quite mad. She told us to come in to the clinic and we heard that we had two weeks to wait for a scan which would reveal whether or not the baby had survived the hormone shut-down caused by my sniffing IVF drugs.

My brain was so screwed with stress and tension that I didn't know what I felt. That must have been the worst two weeks of my life – much worse than the IVF. I thought maybe I should have done the pregnancy test earlier, and I felt guilty that I had waited until four days after my period was due. It made me feel bad that I'd kept the baby without the hormones it needed for an extra four days while I'd sniffed and hadn't done a pregnancy test.

I had injections to give the baby progesterone, and then we just had to wait. That was really sick, because we were half rejoicing that I had conceived, and half realising that we were going to lose our baby. Before, we didn't have a baby to lose because the IVF embryos had never attached themselves. But this one had clung to the womb wall where the others hadn't. Everything had gone the whole way it was meant to go, but I felt I'd just slaughtered it with sniffing for IVF. If the baby had died I don't know where Marcus and I would be now.

Marcus: We didn't know whether to tell anyone or not, because it was both good news and bad news. Because people had been involved in the treatment it wasn't like a normal pregnancy, and it seemed a bit silly to pretend, so we told my Mum and my brothers.

As soon as there was enough to scan they called us in – at that point there would have been a heartbeat. I sat there and the guy behind the screen said, 'Do you want to come over and have a look at your baby?' Then I cried.

Polly: It was stunning to see its heartbeat. All my thoughts were about whether it was alive or dead. I didn't dare imagine what it would be like actually to *look* at my baby.

Marcus: Some people might say we shouldn't ever have bothered with IVF but just let things happen naturally. It wasn't a reality, though. Polly would have been beside herself, and then there would have been the added pressure which could have adversely affected our fertility.

Polly: I don't believe in regret, because I don't believe life can be what it is now without previous events. Everything you go through makes for your current self, and unless you want to dismiss who you are now you shouldn't have regrets.

I feel so exactly like I knew I was going to feel that it isn't terribly exciting. People expect me to jump around all the time, or to be really over the top and over-excited, but I'm not sure I will be. I'll be thrilled to pieces all the time about being pregnant but when you've had some form of disability or handicap or hindrance in life you can get annoyed if people expect you to be bouncing all the time, because you've got what you felt was your right to expect anyway. So yes, I'm really pleased, but I now feel only like I should have done. When you have pain to bear it's enormous and weighty, but when you take pain away you never appreciate that it has gone. For me, contentment and happiness is not being aware that it's particularly brilliant.

Polly gave birth to a baby boy on 30 December 1997.

HELEN AND DARRYL'S STORY

'You look at other people with children who are nine, ten
and eleven, and you should have been having those
children years ago.'

**Helen and Darryl are both in their early forties. Helen is a
home economist and journalist, and Darryl is a tree sur-
geon. They spent some years trying to have a child, and
their daughter was born after their third attempt at IVF.
They are hoping to have another baby, and are about to
start a new round of treatment.**

Darryl: I've never had any doubts I was going to have children.
We thought we'd get married and then we'd go for a baby. We
let it drift on for a few years with nothing happening. We
thought the best way was to get rid of all stress by working
from home. Knowing what we know now, we should have
started earlier.

Helen: I thought something was odd so I went to a clinic. They
sent me for a scan because they thought I had a fibroid. They just
sent me off and said fibroids don't stop you getting pregnant. I
kept thinking that this thing was not right and eventually went
back nearly a year later. I was in a lot of pain. They did another
scan and discovered I'd got an ovarian cyst. I had to go into the
local hospital as an emergency because I think they ruptured it
when they did the scan.

The hospital started investigating my infertility. Really they
just did a blood test and said I wasn't ovulating, so they gave me
Clomid tablets for three months. They did another blood test
and said I was ovulating with the Clomid. But I didn't get
pregnant, so they gave me another three months' worth of
Clomid and then decided to do a laparoscopy.

I regret staying at that hospital. It was just ridiculous. They
would have carried on saying, 'Come back in six months, come
back in six months', and my life would just have disappeared

before me as I saw myself approaching the menopause. I feel I wasted a year there and a year with the cyst when I knew something was wrong even though the doctors kept saying it was all right.

I started reading about infertility and discovered you can't tell from a blood test whether you're ovulating when you take Clomid. So I went to see my GP, who confirmed this, and said he'd refer me to a specialist fertility clinic.

When I first went there I had to pay for another laparoscopy, because they don't necessarily trust what they've been told by another hospital. They also did this horrible womb X-ray. It's the worst thing I've ever had in my life. They put a tube about the size of a ballpoint pen in your cervix and then insert a dye through it into your womb. They let the dye go down your tubes and then X-ray you. It's very uncomfortable when you have it done, but afterwards I was in excruciating pain. They'd said you might get some sort of mild period pain, but I was bedridden. I couldn't move. I'd read somewhere that you could get an awful reaction to the dye. I was convinced I'd got this reaction and rang them up in the morning, but the nurse on the desk said, 'Oh, don't worry, I've had that X-ray done and it's awful. I couldn't move for three days.' It's not very nice, but I suppose they feel it's necessary.

I had to have all that done privately because it speeded things up. It cost about £1,000 for the initial consultancy, the laparo-scopy and the X-ray. That was all all right, and the consultant suggested that I did another couple of cycles of Clomid but they'd scan me to see if it was working. It wasn't, so they had to give me Pergonal, which is one of the injections that they give you when you do IVF to force you to ovulate.

I used to worry about what the Clomid was doing to me. When I got to the Pergonal I thought it was going to work quickly so I didn't worry so much. They don't really seem to know what the drugs do.

The first time with the Pergonal they didn't get the dosage right and it didn't do anything, which made me really tearful and upset because I thought it wasn't going to work. Doctors can be really strange. They are compassionate, but at the same time I think they forget that women get upset. It was a male doctor at the time who was very nice, but he just said, 'It's not working. You're not going to produce any eggs on this amount. We'll have to try again on another occasion.' What he didn't say was, 'Don't worry, we'll get the dosage right.' He obviously wasn't aware of the devastating effect of his bald statement on the women concerned.

The next time they got the dosage too high. They didn't want me to carry on with it because it wasn't an IVF cycle and I had something like fifteen eggs. I had a further three after that when they got the dosage right, but it never worked.

My three Clomid and three Pergonal cycles must have taken about two and a half years, because I used to take breaks between the cycles and I had one long break of about six months because I just thought I'd had enough. I was on the three-year NHS waiting list for IVF anyway, and they suggested I just stick with that.

Helen and Darryl found themselves starting their first IVF attempt soon afterwards.

Darryl: I had no preconceptions about IVF. I just thought I wanted to have a child any way I could. I was pretty ignorant about monthly cycles and so on. It was quite a sharp learning curve to start with.

You're not really informed before you enter into this what it could lead to and what processes you can go for. I think it would be easier if it was actually put down in black and white – your options and what you're going to go through before you actually get to IVF, what the problems could be with you or your partner, and what they're going to try on you. Because you don't know all this you think, 'Why not just go straight for IVF anyway'?
Helen: When you've gone through the first hurdles you think you can't stop because it might be the next thing that works. I don't think by that point I was worried about IVF at all. I just wanted to get on with it and do it. It was all a novelty. I was

excited doing the sniffing and it was OK when I had the injections.

Darryl: I didn't want to give her the injections at all, but in the end I had to. Otherwise it would have meant a whole lot of journeys to the hospital. The first time, the needle went in a couple of millimetres and then sort of hung there.

You have to be a part of it. A lot of women were going to the clinic on their own – their partners weren't there. It's only fair that the man goes through it too – making all the appointments and going together.

Giving your sperm sample, you feel a bit sheepish. Everyone knows where you are going. It was just a bit of a joke really. Apparently with one couple the woman had to go in as well – he couldn't possibly do it on his own. You're all standing outside one after the other. Some are taking five minutes and some are in there half an hour. You think, 'How on earth can it take half an hour?' It's the one operation that most men can cope with.

Helen: The egg collection was fine. They did it under local anaesthetic, but the anaesthetist was really sympathetic and had been topping me up. I was completely out of it. I just heard the odd conversation, nothing very much.

The only traumatic bit was waiting to see if I'd got any embryos afterwards, and that all seemed to go fine. I had fifteen eggs and out of that we got nine embryos.

By that point I was mostly working from home. However, at that particular time I was doing a project for a magazine which meant I had to go into the office three days a week, and it ended up being five days a week. It got really busy at work when I was having the egg collection and embryo transfer. I had a few days off and managed to fit the visits in, and then had to go into work a couple of days after the embryo transfer. I remember being convinced that it was the wrong thing to have done. Maybe it was – I don't know.

When I didn't get pregnant I just thought, 'I've got to do another one now,' and I was desperate to do it almost the next month. But they said we'd have to go back on the NHS waiting list and it would be two or three years before we could have another treatment cycle. We felt that was crazy and decided to pay to go privately. I had to wait a few months, and doing so made me calm down. By the time the moment came round again I was even thinking, 'Do I really want to do this again?' But as soon as I started doing it, it was fine.

Darryl: It's difficult to say whether IVF should be on the NHS – whether someone's heart, hip or lung is more important than someone else's infertility. I think a person waiting for a major operation would say it was worth more than an IVF attempt. Even though we've had IVF both on the National Health and privately, I don't know whether it's fair that it should be available on the NHS. It's very difficult. Should you be allowed to have a set number of IVF attempts before you start having to pay? I don't know.

Helen: When I started treatment I felt quite isolated, and then gradually I met people who were going through fertility treatment of one kind or another or who were having problems and it became more like a club. Quite often I'd go into the unit and see people I knew who'd never told me they were going through IVF and didn't want other people to know.

Usually I did tell people about my own situation. They either said they didn't know how I could go through it all or they were really interested in how things were going and rooting for me to be successful.

Darryl: We didn't go round telling everyone we were going for IVF in a month or anything like that. I wouldn't give them the exact details, though people knew we were doing IVF.

Helen: Darryl never really understood which things upset me and which things didn't. People getting pregnant used to upset me – not people having babies. At first when people told me they were pregnant I sometimes used to hate them because I used to think, 'Why can *you* do it?'

Darryl: I don't think many people are sympathetic to those who can't have children unless they've been through it themselves. If you've had children naturally, one after the other, you don't really think about it. You look at other couples as not having children through choice rather than through medical problems.

Helen: The second egg collection was very painful and I didn't enjoy it at all. The anaesthetist was a particularly insensitive man, and as far as I could gather he just seemed to want it all to be over as quickly as possible. I was the last patient that day. I wasn't even aware the first time that they'd given me a local anaesthetic. The second time I knew about it all right.

Helen and Darryl's second attempt was unsuccessful, and they decided they would try one more treatment cycle.

Darryl: The first time I thought it was going to work, and that was it. When it didn't work the second time I thought we just had to carry on and see what happened. At every point the next stage is difficult. Every stage is a battle and you don't always want to know the results.

Helen: By the time we did the third IVF I'd got to the point where I thought, 'This isn't going to work. I don't even really know why we're bothering. Do I really want to do this again?' It was so nice not to have to do it.

You end up either doing an IVF or waiting to do an IVF. I did find that the break in between them allowed me to forget about it for a while, which was nice. By the time I came round to doing it again I'd think, 'Oh God, here we go again.' And although I'd try not to let it intrude into my life, I couldn't help it doing so.

For the last seven or eight years I'd been thinking about having a baby, actively trying to have a baby and then going through all this fertility treatment. I thought it was ridiculous to keep going on, but having said that I still don't know how I'd have felt if it hadn't worked. We said we'd only do three, but in reality I'm sure I would have done more.

Darryl: I think that third time we were probably going to knock it on the head and give Helen's body a rest for a year or so. It was up to Helen, not up to me. It's not my body that was being jabbed and squeezed. It's easy for a man because you don't really have to do anything, but it's quite a problem having to put your wife or partner through all of that.

Helen: They have a support group at the hospital, which I

joined, but I never went to any meetings. It was only on that last attempt that I actually talked to somebody who happened to be in the waiting room. I still see this girl, and she's a really good friend now.

I had egg collection under general anaesthetic that time, so I didn't know anything about it. It's certainly less traumatic. I always thought I didn't recover particularly well from general anaesthetics, but I did recover reasonably well from this one because for egg collection you're only under for a short time. I was quite sick after the local anaesthetics.

I only had three viable embryos and the hospital said they weren't particularly good quality. Everybody I know who IVF has worked for has said they've been told their embryos weren't particularly good quality. It makes me think the medical people have got it all wrong. Maybe they don't know what good quality is. Because of their poor quality they said they'd put all three embryos back in my womb to give me a better chance. That made me really despondent.

The first two times I had IVF I had this dreadful pain, as if someone was sticking a knife in my stomach, about four days before I started my period. The third time I didn't have that pain, but on the Saturday before I had my blood test I had a really bad period pain. We'd gone to the pictures and I was sitting there squirming around and thinking, 'This hasn't worked again.' When we left I was bawling my eyes out.

I always wanted to get to the day of my blood test without having started my period. Even if I started it in the afternoon I just wanted to get there and have the blood test to see if I had been pregnant. On the Wednesday I still hadn't had my period and I was thinking that for the first time I'd be able to get to the hospital, have a blood test and come home before starting my period. Anyway, I went and had the test. I was in and out of the toilet every five minutes and thought it was nerves, but it was probably the beginning of being pregnant.

They always say they'll ring you with the result between three and five, and I stayed in all afternoon. In fact they didn't ring until half past six, when they said the result was a low positive. I asked what that meant, and they said it was more than likely I'd start my period in the next couple for days. They said it could be an ectopic pregnancy, or that I had a blighted ovum and the pregnancy wasn't going to come to anything, or it could be just a slight blip in the hormone levels and I'd start my period in the next couple of days – but I could be all right.

That weekend we were going to Whitby to stay with some friends, and on the way I kept saying to Darryl, 'You've got to stop the car. I've got to go to the toilet.' I kept thinking that maybe it was working, and then I reminded myself not to be stupid. When I went to bed I had the most excruciating pains all night long, so I just thought I was going to wake up in the morning and find I'd started my period.

The next morning I ate six slices of toast and could have gone on eating more. My friend offered me a cup of coffee and I went, 'Ugh, no thanks.' She said that was the first thing she had gone off when she was pregnant, and she was sure I was pregnant, but I refused to believe her.

We went back home and I still hadn't had my period. I had my second blood test. They said that the results were much better, but it still could all go wrong so I shouldn't get my hopes up too much.

The following week we had to go for our first scan and I was there with the friend I'd met at the clinic. Somebody else went in and came out with a positive result. They'd seen a heartbeat and they'd given her a scan picture. Then my friend went in and I suddenly thought, 'There are three of us here, and the likelihood of all three of us being OK is very small.' I suddenly felt it was all going to go horribly wrong and they were going to tell me there was nothing there. But it turned out to be my friend who had the disappointing news. She was in there for ages – apparently there was a problem with what the scan was showing.

I went in and had my scan and it was all fine, but by then I'd realised something had gone wrong with my friend's, so I asked the staff and they said she had had nothing there. I felt so awful for her, because I'd had this premonition and it turned out to be on her account, not mine.

Darryl: I didn't believe Polly would be here until she was born. You hear so often about people who've gone a long way and still had problems. There can be problems all the way down the line, whether it's an IVF baby or a normal one. I felt that with our luck there was a risk of us having a problem. If you've had to go through IVF to become pregnant you're much more aware of the possibility of another problem arising.

Yet at the maternity clinic you become the same as everyone else. They don't look at you as if you are an IVF couple. As soon as you're there and pregnant you're no one special.

After Helen and Darryl's daughter Polly was born, they hoped they might have another child naturally. They have now decided to try IVF again, and are expecting to start another attempt soon.

Helen: I kept thinking, and I still thought until a couple of months ago, that maybe it would happen on its own. But it never has. Maybe I should have tried earlier. I'm going to see the consultant next month and I think I'll have to wait at least three months. I would have thought that my chances must be better now because of having had a pregnancy, but I don't know. If the original problem is unexplained infertility, maybe once you've had a pregnancy your body is more in tune with it all. Because of my age I suppose they'll have to check my blood for the hormone levels to see whether I'm getting menopausal.

I feel excited in a way about doing it again but I must calm down because it's not going to happen just like that – it never has before. I think I'll give it a year or a year and a half, and try to fit three cycles into that time.

Darryl: We first thought about having children twelve years ago and it took us so long to go through everything, getting more and more desperate. You look at other people with children who are nine, ten and eleven, and you should have been having those children years ago. I don't want to be old when my daughter's in secondary school, but I will be.

We can never go back to the beginning because we've got

Polly now, and I look forward to doing it again knowing that Helen has become pregnant through IVF and the chances are much higher. If a woman has become pregnant and had a baby it must be easier for that programme to run itself over again.

HAYLEY AND CLAUDE'S STORY

'I think I was sold the idea that IVF was the answer to my prayers, but I really didn't know what I was letting myself in for, or how long it could go on for, how many times you have to try and how difficult the whole treatment is.'

Hayley is thirty-five and works in the travel industry. Her husband Claude is an engineer from Quebec in Canada. He is forty-five and has two children from a previous marriage. Hayley and Claude have had five full treatment cycles and three frozen embryo transfers. After their third attempt Hayley discovered she was pregnant, but she miscarried. They are still having treatment.

Hayley: When I was sixteen, I had a lot of fallopian tube infections, and although at that stage the doctors always denied that there would be future repercussions I wasn't terribly convinced. At that time I was very young, and I put it to the back of my mind. I didn't really start thinking about it again until I was about twenty-three, when I was still getting infections too frequently to live with. I went back to the specialists and they said I should have an operation to clear the tubes and see exactly what needed to be sorted out. I would either have to go privately or wait on the NHS list for about two years.

I couldn't carry on taking antibiotics virtually every other month, so I decided to pay to have my tubes sorted out privately. I had the same consultant I would have had under the NHS, but it cost me £2,000. They unblocked the tubes, untwisted them, realigned them and scraped the inside of my womb. There were a lot of adhesions on the tubes, which they sorted out as best they could. They reckoned they'd solved the problem, and you believe them.

A few years later I split up from my then partner. We'd been trying for a baby for about three or four years, and there obviously hadn't been a miraculous cure as the doctors had claimed. They tell you to go away and keep trying, but nothing had happened.

I'd already put myself forward for IVF. Our health authority at the time didn't fund it at all. The only thing you could do was get yourself on the list and they'd eventually send you as a semi-funded patient – you went to the hospital they would have used but paid for it at their rates as opposed to private rates. I was on the list when I met Claude, but it was still too early to think about conceiving so we pushed the appointments back.

Claude: We fell in love very deeply and got involved quickly. Hayley told me within the first month we were together that she would need treatment in order to conceive. She asked me if I'd be willing to go through that and I said I'd have no problem. I wanted to love and cherish a baby again, and I like kids. I was thinking that for me it would be easy. I'd give some samples or specimens, and that would be it.

Hayley: When we did go for the appointment. Claude and I had been together for a while. By that stage I was thirty, and we couldn't afford to wait any longer. We were very secure in our relationship and told them we'd been together for two years – in fact we'd only been together a year.

Hayley and Claude started their first IVF treatment cycle at the hospital soon afterwards.

Hayley: When we went for that first lot of treatment, I produced about forty follicles and had twelve eggs. Then they put the sperm with the eggs. Up until that stage we hadn't had a problem with the sperm count. It was low, but it wasn't so low that they thought it was going to be a problem. But we didn't manage to fertilise any eggs at all at that first attempt.

Claude: I had had no difficulty having kids with my first wife, and I was thinking that for me it would be easy. When they asked me for another sample I started to get nervous. I wasn't aware that my sperm count could be low.

It was normal to start with, and then just deteriorated. I asked why, and they told me it can be what you eat, or it can be stress – various things. They explained that the sperm was produced about eighty days before you ejaculate. When we went for that first treatment cycle we had had a visit from my kids two or three months before, and then my ex-girlfriend came to London and wanted to see me. The stress of the day doesn't matter – it's the stress of the three months before that counts. You don't realise until you start going through this.

When you hear that the sperm has been put with the egg and the outcome wasn't successful, that's when the man stops thinking he has nothing to do and starts to worry.

Hayley: We had a difficult few days relationship-wise, because it was my first IVF treatment. I already knew what the chances were of it actually working, but you try to think it will work first time. Then, when I didn't even get the chance – as far as I was concerned that was it, it was all his fault. I was a complete bitch for a couple of days.

Then you start to get back to normal, stop apportioning blame and begun to think about it logically. It puts a lot of stress on you, and if people were counselled better to start with that might be a way to combat it. We didn't have very much counselling. You just get given a lot of facts and figures, and you're sent off to deal with everything on your own. We were very green back then.

Hayley reacted badly to the drugs on that first attempt.

Hayley: I had very severe hyperstimulation after the treatment. My waist is normally about 23 inches and I was extended to about 33 inches. It was so painful. They didn't do anything for me – they just said take some paracetamol and carry on.

Under normal circumstances I would have taken a week off work sick and not thought about it, but I was going through this training course that I could not miss. I just had to keep going.

Everybody kept asking me what was wrong and I said I'd just had an operation on my stomach. I hadn't been at the job long, so I didn't want to tell everybody the truth because you don't know how that's going to reflect on your work record. I kept it all to myself, but that first week was really awful.

The guy at the hospital was writing a paper on the effects of the drugs and how many people hyperstimulate, and he asked people to come and be monitored. We lived on the coast and I had to keep going back to London every three days, which I had to fit around work as well. It was voluntary, but I hadn't realised how frequently I'd have to go when I agreed to do so.

On that first occasion they had asked us to sign a paper beforehand about what to do with any spare eggs, because they can use them for research purposes. They already knew through the scans that I had loads and loads of follicles, and possibly more eggs than we could utilise. We couldn't freeze at that stage. We said if I produced more than eight eggs they could use some for their own purposes but not for donation. So they tested three eggs with somebody else's sperm. The nurse told me over the phone that the result was positive.

When I went back for another appointment the doctor was surprised that I knew. He said, 'Oh, you shouldn't really have been told about that because it was just a research experiment.' He then said we could use donor sperm next time. We said we'd prefer to carry on with just the two of us, and that knowing that three of my eggs had fertilised was surely a good sign that perhaps next time something would happen.

I was trying to get the doctor to tell me that the eggs were probably OK, but he wouldn't commit himself. The way we saw it, it was more likely to be a problem with the sperm. They told us to come back and try again.

Hayley and Claude went back to the same hospital for a second treatment cycle.

Claude: When we started there was a special room where you go to produce your sample. Everybody is sitting in the corridor, and sometimes there are two or three couples there waiting. You have to walk in front of the people sitting there, pick up the key and go into the room. The key fob is like a piece of plank about a foot long and yellow – you can't miss it. So you're going along the corridor with this great big key and everybody in the hospital knows exactly what it is. You've got to walk as far as the lift, go down a flight to the floor below, back along the corridor and then disappear into this little room for however long it takes you. Some men take ten minutes, some half an hour. Meanwhile there are lots of people waiting outside to see doctors in another department altogether. It's so indiscreet it's untrue. And when you're in there and somebody knocks on the door it's something else . . .

Apparently what you eat and what you wear could make a difference to whether or not you are fertile. You have to let your body breathe, so it's not good if you wear jeans that are too tight or anything like that. And stress isn't good for your sperm count – it could be work, anything like that. So you have to make sure that you are in good health, keep fit and think about it every day, even if you know you won't be giving a sample next week. If you keep on form you'll be ready.

So now I have the stress of keeping fit all the time, of making sure I'm not doing things I shouldn't! I think about what I'm wearing and eating more than I did before, and I try to keep my system working normally.

Hayley: You do try to adhere to all these different things, but at first you don't know what you're letting yourself in for – like all the drugs you have to take. The job I was doing made it very difficult to sniff regularly every four hours, so I chose injections which meant once every twelve hours. I don't mind doing them myself at home.

Claude: At the beginning I was doing the injections because I said I wanted to do something and to be part of it, but Hayley prefers to do it herself. Now I just prepare them. But one day I prepared the wrong injection – it was a simple mistake. You think it's nothing – just an injection to produce some eggs – but it could be dangerous.

Hayley: He gave me the Profasi instead of the Pergonal. I was in tears and we were both panicking. We phoned the hospital and we were told to stop that cycle and start again. There are lots of things that you think you're learning as you go along, and then one little mistake and you're back to square one.

On the second occasion I again produced loads of follicles, and about nine or ten eggs. Eight fertilised and we managed to have one treatment plus two frozen embryo implants, one of which we had done at a private hospital because by that stage we'd decided we weren't very keen on the NHS hospital.

After their second unsuccessful attempt Hayley and Claude were losing faith in the hospital where they were being treated.

Claude: When I went the first time and I was waiting in the corridor to give a sample, I was shocked. It's not the cleanest of places, and I didn't feel very comfortable. The standards of hospitals in Canada are higher than they are in the UK – more like a private hospital here. I felt they could make a mistake very easily. I sometimes feel as if we're having the wrong embryos transferred. It's possible, you know.

Some time ago we got a phone call from them asking us what we wanted to do with the embryos we had frozen in storage there. Since we knew we had no frozen embryos left we were shocked. Then we started thinking that if there were still two frozen embryos belonging to us, they must have given us some-one else's a few months ago. We called the hospital, and they said the secretary had made a mistake, but I'm not convinced. I would be more worried but I saw the way they kept the files, and also because it's a teaching hospital the staff often change. It doesn't give you much confidence in the hospital, or hope. If they're getting things like that wrong, whatever else is wrong?

Hayley: We also felt that they didn't treat you well, particularly after we'd been to the private hospital and had the frozen embryo transfer there, where they make you lie down for a couple of hours afterwards. I'm not saying that doing so will necessarily mean that any of the embryos will take, but it boosts your confidence when you feel they're really taking care.

Claude: At the private hospital they receive you in a room, and you have a cup of tea, and then they take you down to the theatre on a stretcher. It's totally professional. At the teaching hospital you sit waiting in a corridor until it's your turn. You jump on the bed, and then it's finished.

Hayley and Claude decided to have their next treatment cycle at another private hospital, where they felt the treatment would be better.

Hayley: You felt that they had more time for you, that you weren't rushed in and rushed out. You were given time to ask questions without feeling that you were keeping somebody else waiting. And collecting the eggs was done differently – you get on a stretcher and they take you down in a proper gown, rather than just taking your bottom half off and sticking your legs in the air.

On one occasion at the NHS hospital the egg collection was so painful I said they had to give me a breather. I asked for some more anaesthetic, but they said, 'No, no. You've had enough.' I kept saying I hadn't. I'm not somebody who flinches at a bit of pain, but this was really bad and it took a long time because I always produce so many follicles, all of which have to be drained. I just couldn't stand it. At the private hospital I had only one bad moment. There was one particularly difficult follicle which was in the wrong position, and the doctor couldn't get the needle there. That was the only time I flinched throughout the whole process. If they could do that there, why can't they do it elsewhere?

Claude: You can feel that it's painful and I don't like it happening at all, but I want to be there. It's one of the ways I can feel involved. Even if it's only a scan, I do my best to take time off work to be there. I have no reason to be there for a scan, but it's something we have to do together. I want to do everything I can.

The egg collection is done with a syringe and you can follow it on the scan picture. It's unbelievable.

At the NHS hospital, you didn't know who was going to be there. Every time you had a collection it was done by different people whom you had first met five minutes before in a corridor. At the private hospital the doctor who saw Hayley to start with was the doctor who did the collection and everything. He was there all the time.

Hayley: You didn't have the same person at the teaching hospital, so it lacked continuity. They had to look at the file every time they said anything or every time you said anything. At the private hospital they already knew who you were, they knew what they'd done and what drugs you'd been on because everybody reacts differently to them and has to take a bit more or a bit less. They were more aware of each patient as an individual.

Hayley and Claude's third attempt at IVF was followed by a positive pregnancy test.

Hayley: Once the IVF had worked, the last thing that I expected was to miscarry. I know it's something you should look at because the percentages are very high, but once I was pregnant that was it as far as I was concerned. I'm not saying they should make women more aware of the possibility of miscarriage, because perhaps that's too much to cope with before you start on IVF.

At about eight or nine weeks we knew there was a problem. My scan at six weeks was fine, but when I went back for the second scan there was no heartbeat. You could see the sac, but it wasn't growing any more.

At that stage they offered to have me in and do a D & C, but I said I'd rather miscarry naturally. My GP said it would just be like a bad period, and I thought I'd be laid up for a couple of days, take a few strong painkillers and be all right. But it was absolutely awful – far worse than a bad period.

It started at about ten in the evening. At midnight I told Claude I couldn't handle it any more, so we went to casualty. I was wheeled straight into one of their little cubicles, because they could see I was as pale as a sheet and in severe pain. I told

the nurse I was miscarrying and she said she'd call the doctor. I
kept sending Claude out to get the nurse because I needed
painkillers, but she wouldn't give me anything until the doctor
had seen me. Claude felt bad because he couldn't do anything.
The doctor came after about two hours, and he still wouldn't
give me anything until the gynaecologist had seen me. The
gynaecologist didn't turn up for four hours, by which time I
was actually coming through the worst of it.

The nurse gave me a bedpan to do a urine sample and I felt this
thing plop out. I was petrified. I expected a few blood clots but
not this mass of a thing to come out. I looked in the bedpan and I
thought I was losing my insides. I had no idea it was going to be
like that.

When I look back on it I realise I was having contractions. It's
obviously not like a birth, but to start with the pain was
intermittent and then it was there constantly, just pulling at you.

I just kept thinking, 'Why me?' which is what you think
anyway before all this rigmarole. I know that for any woman
a miscarriage is a bad time, but for me it was worse because I
couldn't just go home, wait until the next period and try again. It
meant going through the whole process again. But I did start to
think that at least I *could* fall pregnant. It's just a question of
giving it another go and another go and another go until things
work. The experience did give us a lot of positive thoughts as
well.

Apart from my family, who knew I was going through the
treatment, I'd really only told one or two close friends at work, so
I didn't have that many people to explain to. They didn't know
what to say to me, and I didn't want to make them feel bad or
embarrassed.

**Hayley and Claude have since had two more unsuccessful
IVF treatment cycles and are continuing with their treatment.**

Hayley: To start with I wasn't very open with people about
going through IVF, apart from very close friends. Now I tend to

be a lot more open because it isn't anything to be ashamed of. People are asking, 'You're thirty-five – aren't you thinking of having kids?' Do you lie or do you tell them the truth? Most people's reactions are really good. They're very sympathetic and try to be as supportive as they can. But a lot of people are totally unaware.

Claude: Socially, it's now become more acceptable. We open the paper and nearly every week there's a story about IVF or something similar, because it's getting more and more common. But the average person is not aware of what it is or what it involves. The GPs are also not aware of the kind of support they need to give their patients, because they don't have a clue about what you actually have to face.

Hayley: I've changed GPs about three times. You ask your doctor to prescribe you the drugs the hospital have requested, and the doctor asks what they are for. The first GP said he didn't know if he could prescribe them because I was under his care, and if anything happened while I was on the drugs it would be his fault if he'd prescribed them. I said it's all in consultation with the hospital, and it's not as if they're banned drugs.

A lot of people still don't know what IVF stands for. Then you have to say you suffer from infertility, and the treatment you go through is IVF which stands for in vitro fertilisation. And they say, 'What?', and you say, 'Test-tube babies', and then it falls into place.

That television programme *Making Babies* showed a lot more people the reality of what happens. Before then, most people assumed that if you needed IVF you went in, it worked first time and off you went. The publicity has done us good, because it means we don't have to explain quite so much any more.

We set up a support group with a few other people in our town. We started with four or five of us, and in the end there were about fifteen or twenty. It's not until you talk to people that you realise how many have difficulties of one sort or another. It helped a lot of people, particularly those who were going through their first treatments or hadn't embarked on any treatment yet. It gave them a really good idea of what to expect and how you react to the drugs, and of all the variations of treatment.

I get PMT anyway, but I don't usually lose my temper. On the drugs I could feel myself getting ratty, and it was definitely a side-effect of them rather than what I'm normally like. When you talk to other people you get their reactions, and it helps the men to understand that it's not just their hysterical partners who aren't coping with it very well – it really does have an effect on your emotional outlook. I could be fine at work because I knew I had to keep everything at bay. But because you are doing that for hours on end five days a week, by the time you get home you're even worse. I work with customers and I can't afford to have tantrums, so Claude has to put up with double the frustration at the end of the day. But you learn to live with it, and if we do have an argument I'll say, 'It's the drugs, it's not me.' Probably sometimes it really is me, but it's very difficult to decide which is which.

By the time we set up the group I was one of the most experienced because I'd already been through quite a lot of treatment. I could tell new members things that you just don't think to ask the doctors. Now I write my questions down on a pad as soon as I think of them and I take the pad in with me, because otherwise I get in there and forget and don't get answers to half the things I meant to.

Hayley and Claude have been considering other options.

Claude: I'm a planning type, whereas Hayley is more easy-going. I said I didn't mind if we went on trying for ever – we don't have a problem with money or anything – but we should also think about something else such as a surrogate mother or adoption. We came to the conclusion that adoption would not be easy for us in this country, because of the way it's dealt with by the authorities. The fact that I'm not English and she's younger than me could cause a lot of problems.

Hayley: If you have so many failures you have to think about alternatives. Although I've had enough of the ups and downs of it, even more important is the fact that time is marching on and neither of us is getting any younger. Claude's forty-five, I'm thirty-five. I could carry on for another ten years, but that makes him fifty-five. I think I was sold the idea that IVF was the answer to my prayers, but I really didn't know what I was letting myself in for, or how long it could go on for, how many times you have to try and how difficult the whole treatment is.

We've got another frozen embryo one to go for, after which I'll probably go back again and have another bash. I hope I'll produce as many eggs again, so we've got another couple of frozen attempts. But I think that will probably be my lot for this way of doing things.

After that I might think of surrogacy with my egg. It depends on what happens between now and then. Two of my girlfriends have offered to be surrogates. I wouldn't say yes automatically, but whether we accept or not it's really nice to think that a friend would do that for you. We'd have to go through the counselling and make sure that we were completely aware of what we'd be letting ourselves in for, but it's a road I would consider going down because genetically the baby would still be ours.

Claude: It would be another stressful situation. When I read a story recently about a surrogate mother who decided not to give the baby back to a couple I was shocked, because it's not fair. I put myself in the position of the couple who wanted the baby. That's a situation you risk getting into.

For me it would be really difficult if the surrogate mother lived miles away so that you'd be unable to see her often or have contact with her and give her support. I think I would miss something about the pregnancy.

Hayley: It's a difficult path to go down. Perhaps I have too rosy a view of how straightforward it could be.

We've already had so many attempts. A line has to be drawn at some stage. I think I'd probably give it until I'm forty, which is another five years. After however many attempts I'd fit into that period of time I will have had enough.

NICKY AND JACKIE'S STORY

'I was sure that if anybody knew I was a lesbian they wouldn't agree to pay for me to have surgery to see if I was infertile. They'd say why should I have a baby anyway?'

Nicky and Jackie have been together for seven years. Jackie has been married and has two school-age children, Becky and Tom, from that relationship. Nicky wanted to have a child of her own, but found she wasn't getting pregnant when they tried insemination with donor sperm. Eventually they sought medical help, and their son Alexander was born after their first IVF attempt.

Nicky: When I was eleven I was seriously ill with a burst appendix, or peritonitis. I came across a book in the school library which said peritonitis could be a cause of infertility. But I'd always known that I wanted a baby, and always imagined that I would have one.

When Jackie and I first got together we discussed the fact that I would want a baby at some point. We decided to start trying, and we went to a group for women who wanted to get pregnant through donor sperm. They advertised for sperm donors and had a file of donors. We looked through the papers and chose a guy called Tim. Our main criterion was health – he must be tested for every conceivable transmittable disease.

Jackie: Tim was also a donor at the Pregnancy Advisory Service, and we thought that was good because he'd definitely be tested. There was lots of information in the papers – details about the colour of hair and eyes, and whether the men were in relationships – but no photographs. At that point we didn't want involvement from the father, but we did want the child to know the father so there would be some identity.

Nicky: We very naively met him and decided to go for a meal. It was quite an intimate sort of restaurant. Within minutes we knew that we would never have him as a donor, but we still had to sit through the whole dinner. That was a disaster.

Jackie: He was asking questions that weren't appropriate – questions about our relationship.

Nicky: There were certain things that definitely worried us about him. He did have a girlfriend, but he hadn't told her that he was a sperm donor. There were other things, too, that suggested he wasn't very stable, not sorted out. We just thought he didn't suit us at all.

The next stage was asking around our friends. We decided to go for a gay man who wanted to be a donor and perhaps an involved father too. We didn't want a straight man, because if he got into a stable heterosexual relationship he might fight for custody of the child.

A friend who is gay suggested a guy called John. We went round for dinner and he seemed very charming and attractive. We thought it might work out.

Jackie: He wanted the level of involvement that we were keen on. He didn't want too much, but he did want a bit.

Nicky: We started trying with him, using his fresh sperm. The first time we did it we sterilised things with tablets. That would kill anything. Later we'd just rinse out a yoghurt pot with warm water. He did his sample into that, and then we'd just syringe it up. You think it's all got to be done in such a precious way, but sperm can last for forty-eight hours at room temperature.

Jackie: We found out lots of information, like there was no point using a glass container to collect the sperm. The sperm heads stick to the glass and they get lost. You have to use plastic – hence the yoghurt pot.

Nicky: I'd been taking my temperature for months in preparation for this, but there was no pattern. Then we started using ovulation test kits, which I used to spend a fortune on because my cycle is hugely irregular – anything from seventeen to fifty days.

Either John would come to us or we'd go to him. We only wanted to do it with both of us there, and there was a difficulty with the distances involved. Sometimes I'd have to drive over to him and collect the sample, transfer it to a syringe and then drive over to Jackie's and inseminate there.

We did it with him for six or seven months, and it didn't work. He'd obviously had all the health tests before, but then he went for a sperm analysis. It came back showing that some of them were dead and the rest were swimming the wrong way. Although his fertility wasn't hopeless, it wasn't the best. On top of that was the fact that, although we talked a lot about safe sex and he said he was going to practise it, he was going out to bars and meeting people and having sex with them. I was worried. There's hardly any research on whether you can transmit HIV between women and I could take the risk for me, but how could I put Jackie at risk? It's like having sex with the highest-risk group you possibly could. We couldn't take that risk.

Nicky and Jackie decided they couldn't carry on using John's sperm, and looked for another way to find a suitable donor.

Nicky: We went to the Pregnancy Advisory Service, where we were able to be totally 'out'. In fact they'd treated some other lesbians that we know. You'd just go to the clinic and it would be anonymous sperm.

Jackie: They gave us counselling and they assessed Nicky. They did blood tests and medical tests, and they were assessing her all the time because they wanted a record. If she didn't get pregnant they wanted to know why.

Nicky: They did a hormone test to see if I was ovulating, and they thought I was so they said we should give it six months. They were able to keep a medical account of what was going on, and to help me with the ovulation bit. I'd do the test with a kit, and then I'd ring them and say, 'I think today's the day.' I'd go up there and they'd double-check by examining the mucus and my cervix. They sometimes sent me away and said it wasn't the right day, and I'd have to go back maybe three or four days in a row. We'd try to go together whenever possible.

Jackie: They showed me the sperm all whizzing about under the microscope. Although it was anonymous they let you know things like the colour of hair and eyes, height and tone of skin of the donor. We ordered some that was very similar to Nicky's hair colour and skin tone.

Nicky: We saw the consultant at the beginning and again after six months, and they were getting more and more concerned about the peritonitis. I've got quite a lot of scars, and they could see it had been a serious operation. They said I had to get it checked out, which meant a laparoscopy. For this I had to ask my GP to refer me to a hospital.

All the time I was uptight about involving doctors, because I wasn't 'out' to my GP. But I was going for a smear at the local hospital, and the consultant there was very friendly and positive. I explained the situation and she said I could write a self-referral letter to a women's hospital, not even bothering to go to the GP. I was sure that if anybody knew I was a lesbian they wouldn't agree to pay for me to have surgery to see if I was infertile. They'd say why should I have a baby anyway?

I wrote a letter anyway, and they replied and said they'd see me. I saw a consultant from hell – very traditional, bow-tied. I went on my own because we were so het up that people wouldn't give us surgery if we told them our true situation. I'm sure husbands were mentioned and he was calling me 'Mrs', and I just went along with that.

He said that he'd do the laparoscopy. I remember vividly asking if he could say what would happen and what the risks were. His answer was: 'I'm the sort of consultant who chooses to tell my patients as little as possible, and I'm certainly not going to give a textbook explanation.' I felt so belittled, so small and vulnerable. I came out virtually in tears.

On the day of the operation I was terrified that somebody was going to find out I didn't have a husband. Jackie came with me. I had the pre-med and I was getting hazier and hazier. I was suddenly surrounded by all these specialists asking if my husband had had sperm tests, who his GP was, and did I know I could get pregnant even if my husband only had one sperm. I was so frightened and confused and I was telling everybody different things. I didn't know what I was saying.

Jackie: First of all Nicky said her husband had left her, and then she talked about him being killed in a car crash.

Nicky: I went down for the operation, and as I was coming round there was this woman on the bed next to me and she'd just come up from theatre. She said she'd had a laparoscopy, and they couldn't see what was wrong with her because she was too fat.

We went back to hear what they'd found, and the doctor said he was sorry but according to the notes they hadn't been able to see anything at all because I was obese. Then he looked at me and said, 'You don't look obese.' I told him about the woman who'd said she'd been too fat for them to discover anything. It seemed they'd managed to muddle up our notes.

I said I had to see the person who had done the surgery, and they went off and got the consultant. He said they had found fatty adhesions around both ovaries – they were totally en-meshed. One was slightly worse than the other. He described it as a bit like being in a plastic bag, and I asked if there were any holes in the plastic bag for the eggs to get out. He said, 'Maybe', but he didn't sound very hopeful. Then he told me to come in for major surgery which might clear the adhesions.

Jackie: That carried a risk of greater infertility, so we went back to the Pregnancy Advisory Service and they suggested we went to this private fertility clinic as an alternative. There they would rinse the sperm through to leave only the swimmers and not the ocean, and they also had a different technique of inserting the sperm much higher, through the cervix, called intra-uterine insemination. So we went there and the doctor was lovely.

Nicky: She said, 'Why don't you try IVF? Why are you thinking of major surgery when IVF is the best way of getting pregnant? Why are you thinking of trying intra-uterine insemination? Let's just skip all those steps and go straight for IVF.'

We said we thought IVF was for people who were in their late forties and desperate, but she said no. It was just good to hear the news.

It cost £3,000 because it was a private clinic, and I asked if there was any way we could get the treatment on the NHS. She told us about a self-funding programme at a fertility unit at a nearby hospital.

Jackie: She gave us the details of the department and wrote a referral letter. She was really helpful – she just wanted Nicky to be pregnant.

Nicky: There were certain people we met who were just incredibly helpful, like the woman at our local hospital who did the smear. She put us on to the women's hospital, and that was the only bad experience. The private clinic and the fertility unit were so helpful. No one had a problem with the fact that it was two women trying to have a baby.

We saw a really good consultant at the fertility unit – a wonderful, very open-minded person. We just walked in there and she said, 'So you're lesbians.' We usually leave it for a while before we say that. We talked to her about how to get hold of the drugs. The self-funding programme meant we'd pay them £900 for their expertise and equipment, but that didn't include the drugs. For that I had to go back to my GP to see if I could get them on the NHS. She didn't think there would be a problem, but I said I wasn't happy about coming 'out' to the GP – it was too much of a risk.

Jackie: I rang the GP's practice and said I was thinking of moving into the area. I explained I was in a relationship with a woman and wanted to do IVF, and asked if they would fund the drugs if they took me on as a patient. They said they'd fund single women for IVF, but not women in same-sex relationships.

Nicky: I rang the local health authority and they said the same. It's their policy. They pay for single women, but not lesbians.

Then I had to go down to the GP. She asked about husbands and things, and I just went along with it. I never knew whether she knew that I haven't got a husband.

Nicky's doctor agreed to prescribe the drugs she would need for the IVF cycle, but she and Jackie had to decide whether they wanted to use an anonymous donor sperm at the hospital or to find a known donor.

Nicky: We tried a little bit more to get a father involved. All the people we asked were gay and either they just couldn't handle the idea because they wanted to live with the child, or they never discussed it and wouldn't get back to us. Finally we decided we didn't really want an involved father anyway. Why have a third person when it was going to be so complicated?

We had to pay £90 for donor sperm at the hospital. We got happier and happier with the idea, although we had reservations about it. I don't know how difficult it's going to be as Alexander gets older. That's a problem we'll have to deal with. The same donor has got three more samples stored so we can have three more goes. I pay £50 a year to keep it there, and they'll store it for five years.

We had counselling before the treatment, but it was really just checking to see what we would say to the baby about how it had come into the world, and all those things. They also wanted to know how physical we would be in front of the child. I got really embarrassed – it wasn't easy to answer.

Jackie: We just said that we'd be the same as most heterosexual people. Just a quick hug, a quick peck, that's about it.

Nicky: We'd had counselling before, at the Pregnancy Advisory Service, which I felt was to see whether we were going to give the right answers. It did help us to think about things, but I believe they would have hesitated about taking us on if we'd said we'd tell the baby that his father had died or something like that.

At the hospital they were a bit more interested in our feelings. They wanted to contact both our GPs to see if we were mentally stable enough to be parents. We weren't 'out' to our GPs, so in the letters they wrote we just said that Jackie was going to be a guardian to the baby.

Jackie: They were asking if we wanted a baby to save our relationship, or to build the relationship. It felt very testing, but it was done as sensitively as it could be.

I was surprised we'd got so far. Each time we were surprised at how far we'd got, and that we'd had such positive feedback. By that time we decided we were going to be totally honest because we were just getting into more and more of a mess when we weren't able to be so.

Nicky: When we'd lied at the women's hospital it had been really bad for both of us. I've never felt so vulnerable as when I was about to go down to theatre and they'd got this whole lie. It didn't feel good. If somebody's going to chop you up you want them to know who you are.

Eventually Nicky and Jackie were told they could start their first treatment cycle.

Nicky: We got the OK, and we went to see a nurse. When I'm anxious I keep interrupting people constantly. She was trying to tell me what order to take the drugs in, and how to do it. I kept saying, 'But . . . but . . .' and she told me to shut up.

One of my hormone levels was high, which meant they would have to give me the highest level of drugs to get the ovaries stimulated. If it didn't work there wasn't much they could do, because my hormones were like those of a much older person.

I didn't do the nasal spray. It would have meant sniffing quite a few times during the day and I'd be in meetings and so on. The injections were just twice a day, twelve hours apart, which I did at eight in the morning and at eight at night. I was absolutely obsessed. I went off and bought a watch with an alarm that would go off at eight every morning and eight every night. I was very concerned about the temperature the drugs had to be kept at. We were still living in separate places and we both had ancient fridges, so I went and bought a fridge thermometer.

Nicky and Jackie decided that Nicky would do the first-stage injections herself, and Jackie would do all the others.

Nicky: I had to inject myself at the hospital the first time. They wanted to see that I could do it, and I was really scared. I found it difficult to put that first needle in – it's very thin. The nurse was very supportive and told me my tummy was the best place to do it. I found that idea horrendous, but eventually I realised it was nothing. I actually found it best to do it on my thigh. You do end up with lots of little bits of bruising.

Jackie: I had to practise injections on an orange, injecting it with water at the hospital. The first time I did it for real I was quite scared, but it was OK. Then it got a bit more difficult. Nicky became more and more relaxed, but psychologically it became more and more difficult for me. I was really surprised, because beforehand I was looking forward to doing the injections.

Nicky: I was living at my house, but spending most of my time at Jackie's. Every morning the children would see me injecting. Often they'd say, 'Wait for me', because they wanted to come and look. They knew the whole story, and they'd been involved right from the beginning. They've got a really good understanding of what it is that we did.

We were really surprised that you had to mix up your own phials of drugs to make the solution for the injections. I'd line them all up and I was really worried about the cats jumping on the table or somebody knocking it. Becky and Tom would help Jackie set the phials up, snapping the tops off.

Jackie: We were really calm and supportive to each other. We just went through it very systematically. It seemed very easy and I didn't ever feel excluded. We'd go to scans together. Nicky would just say, 'Can my friend come in?'

We didn't go to the hospital self-help group because we didn't feel confident that there would be many people in our situation. We felt quite vulnerable anyway, and we didn't want to expose ourselves further.

Nicky: There wasn't anything about it in books. You'd go to the pregnancy section in bookshops and realise that what you were looking for wasn't there. I'd feel really embarrassed when I went to the assistants to say I was looking for a book on infertility, especially when they fumbled around and didn't know where to find one.

Jackie: They'd shout out, 'Infertility . . . where are the infertility books?' At least that was what it felt like.

Nicky: We did buy two books, but they weren't specifically about IVF. There was just a small chapter about it among all the other processes you could go through.

Despite the concerns about Nicky's hormone levels, the first stages of the cycle went well enough for them to go on to egg collection.

Nicky: Before you go in for the egg collection you're meant to choose some music that you like. We chose a song I really liked by Everything but the Girl. You take a painkiller the night before and then they give you pethidine. I was a bit disappointed really because I was so out of it, but Jackie watched the collection.

Jackie: It was terrible, because Nicky was in a lot of pain and crying. They were telling her to take deep breaths, but she wouldn't do it and was doing shallow breathing. They were getting quite impatient with her. I think you have to relax for the needle to move around.

They had two screens – I could see one and they were working from the other one. You just see them point to the follicles and scoop them out.

Nicky: Six or seven eggs fertilised. They wanted to put three embryos back, but we didn't want triplets. They talked about embryo reduction – selective termination of one or more embryos – if three had taken. We read up about triplets and said we'd go for two embryos this time and then decide what to do after that. I talked to friends who had twins and decided that it would be crazy – but crazily good. They showed us both the embryos on the closed-circuit screen before they put them back in, and they said they were good because all the cells were symmetrical.

I don't think we were worried about anything because it was our first go, and we were just excited that we'd done the cycle. We weren't thinking that it was going to work. Everything was good news – yes, they'd got eggs; yes, they'd fertilised; and yes, they were able to put two good ones in. This was the biggest chance that we'd ever had, so we had great hopes.

We went away and it was obviously on our minds. I was constantly thinking my period had started and going off to the loo. I'm the sort of person who's never sure whether it's started or not. I wondered what would happen if I found out it hadn't worked and I was at the office and Jackie wasn't there. Should I just go straight home or what? It was news that concerned both of us, and I didn't want to tell someone else at work first. I was at work during the whole cycle, but I spoke to my boss before I started and she was really good. I wanted her to know what was going on in case I needed to rush off.

You were meant to wait sixteen days before doing a test, but on the fifteenth day we couldn't wait any longer. We did a test, and it was negative. But even so I was still saying that I knew I wasn't going to have a period. Jackie said when she was pregnant she could tell right from the start, but I never felt I was in touch with whatever that is. At the same time another bit of me couldn't imagine having another period for a long time.

We could have done another test twenty-four hours later, but we said we'd wait for five days. That's when we did it, and it came out positive. It was amazing. We rang the hospital and ten days later we went for a scan and saw our baby. We saw him at four cells, then as a blob, and then at twenty weeks. For me, the scans are a really important part of the bonding.

Until we had IVF there was no way my eggs could have got down into the tubes – they could never have met any sperm. The consultant said it was as if the ovaries were encased in chewing gum, and the eggs could never get out. I guess that's why we were quite positive about IVF – it was going to be the first proper chance of sperm meeting egg. Most people don't know for certain that they haven't met somewhere along the line, but we knew they couldn't do that and it made it feel very different.

There was nothing negative about the IVF. It was really amazing. Some of the other stuff was really hard to go through, but the IVF was very easy for us. I had a discussion with the consultant and said I'd felt fine, that the drugs didn't affect me and it had all been very calm and straightforward. She said it could be for some women. There's no guarantee it would be like that again, and I think we were really lucky. The day after Alexander was born Jackie said, 'Would you go through all that again?', and I said yes.

Glossary

Adhesions: tissue which sticks organs together. For example, uterine adhesions means that the walls of the womb are stuck together.

Blood pressure, raised: blood pressure is monitored regularly during pregnancy as high blood pressure can be a sign of pre-eclampsia (see below).

Braxton Hicks contractions: weak contractions which occur in late pregnancy as a practice for labour.

Congenital: dating from birth.

D&C: dilatation and curettage. This is a common surgical procedure during which the cervix is opened and the inside of the womb is scraped. It may be used after a miscarriage to clear the womb.

Fibroid: benign growth which is found in the uterus.

Gamete: a sperm or egg.

HRT: Hormone Replacement Therapy. HRT is used to help alleviate menopausal symptoms by replacing the hormones which decline at this time.

Induction: induction of labour involves artificially starting labour by breaking the waters and using drugs to stimulate contractions.

Low birthweight: a baby weighing less than 2.5 kilograms is usually considered to have a low birthweight and may need special care. A low birthweight baby may have difficulty feeding or breathing, and be more susceptible to infection.

Menopause (premature): the average age for the menopause is around 50, but some women have a premature menopause and stop ovulating at a much younger age. In such circumstances the only way to get pregnant is to use a donated egg.

Oedema: swelling. During pregnancy it is quite common for feet, hands or ankles to swell.

Pituitary gland: a gland at the base of the brain which is responsible for hormone production.

Placenta: attached to wall of the womb, the placenta provides a support system for a growing baby.

Pre-eclampsia: pre-eclampsia, or pregnancy-induced hypertension, is a complication which can occur during pregnancy. Symptoms usually include high blood pressure, swelling of feet, hands or ankles and protein in the urine.

Rubella: German measles. If caught in early pregnancy, German measles can cause malformations in the baby.

Sac (amniotic): bag of waters in which an embryo floats.

Thyroid: problems with the thyroid gland, which is situated in the neck, can in rare cases be the cause of failure to ovulate.

Zygote: a fertilised egg.

Useful Addresses

Human Fertilisation and Embryology Authority
Paxton House
30 Artillery Lane
London E1 7LS
Tel: 0171 377 5077

ISSUE
114 Lichfield Street
Walsall WS1 1SZ
Tel: 01922 722888

CHILD
Charter House
43 St Leonards Road
Bexhill-on-Sea
East Sussex TN40 1JA
Tel: 01424 732361

DI Network
PO Box 265
Sheffield S3 7YX
Tel: 0181 245 4369

Dalsy Chain (Premature menopause self-help network)
PO Box 2829
Blandford Forum
Dorset DT11 8NZ

NEEDS (National Egg and Embryo Donation Society)
St Mary's Hospital
Whitworth Park
Manchester M13 0JH
Tel: 0161 276 6000

Miscarriage Association
c/o Clayton Hospital
Northgate
Wakefield
West Yorkshire WF1 3JS
Tel: 01924 200799

TAMBA (Twins & Multiple
 Births Association)
PO Box 30
Little Sutton
South Wirral L66 1TH
Tel: 0151 348 0020

COTS (Childlessness
 Overcome Through
 Surrogacy)
Loandhu Cottage
Gruids
Lairg
Sutherland IV27 4EF
Tel: 01549 402401

**British Agencies for
 Adoption and Fostering**
Skyline House
200 Union Street
London SE1 0LX
Tel: 0171 593 2000

OASIS (Overseas Adoption
 Support and Information
 Services)
Dan y Craig
Balaclava Road

Glais
Swansea SA7 9HJ
Tel: 01792 844329

British Acupuncture Council
Park House
206–208 Latimer Road
London W10 6RE
Tel: 0181 964 0222

The Society of Homeopaths
2 Artizan Road
Northampton NN1 4HU
Tel: 01604 621400

**Aromatherapy Organisations
 Council**
3 Latymer Close
Braybrooke
Market Harborough
Leicestershire LE16 8LN
Tel: 01858 434242

**National Association of
 Medical Herbalists**
56 Longbrook St.
Exeter
Devon EX4 6AH
Tel: 01392 426022

Index